Changing Body Composition through Diet and Exercise

Michael J. Ormsbee, Ph.D.

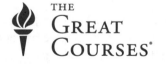

THE
GREAT
COURSES®

PUBLISHED BY:

THE GREAT COURSES
Corporate Headquarters
4840 Westfields Boulevard, Suite 500
Chantilly, Virginia 20151-2299
Phone: 1-800-832-2412
Fax: 703-378-3819
www.thegreatcourses.com

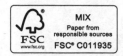

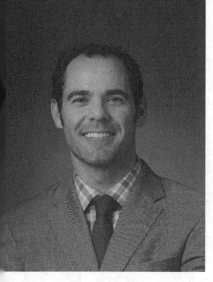

Michael J. Ormsbee, Ph.D.
Assistant Professor in Nutrition, Food, and Exercise Sciences
Florida State University

D
r. Michael J. Ormsbee is an Assistant Professor in the Department of Nutrition, Food, and Exercise Sciences and the Interim Director for the Institute of Sports Sciences and Medicine at Florida State University (FSU). He is a faculty affiliate of the Center for Advancing Exercise and Nutrition Research on Aging and the Institute for Successful Longevity at FSU. Dr. Ormsbee is also an Honorary Research Fellow at the University of KwaZulu-Natal in Durban, South Africa. He earned his B.S. in Exercise Science and Business from Skidmore College, his M.S. in Exercise Physiology and Sports Nutrition from South Dakota State University, and his Ph.D. in Bioenergetics from East Carolina University. Dr. Ormsbee's research and expertise involve the interaction of exercise, nutrition, and supplementation to achieve optimal body composition, human performance, and health in both athletes and clinical populations.

Prior to arriving at FSU, Dr. Ormsbee taught and conducted research at Skidmore College. His major research contributions have included investigation into meal composition and frequency, exercise type and duration, nighttime feeding, and the use of supplements to alter body composition and performance. Dr. Ormsbee started Ormsbee Fitness Consulting in 2006 and has worked with everyone from Olympic athletes to everyday people. He is a sought-after speaker both nationally and internationally on issues related to exercise, diet, and performance nutrition.

While at FSU, Dr. Ormsbee won the 2013–2014 University Teaching Award, the Excellence in Online Course Design Award, the Excellence in Online Teaching Award, and the 2013 Transformation through Teaching Award. He was also selected for the Guardian of the Flame Faculty Award by the Burning Spear leadership honor society in 2015. In 2012, Dr. Ormsbee was elected as a Fellow of the International Society of Sports Nutrition, and in 2014, he was elected as a Fellow of the American College of Sports Medicine.

Dr. Ormsbee regularly publishes his research in the top scientific journals in his field and presents at national and international conferences. He is active in education and outreach, giving seminars to academics, athletes, and the public. Dr. Ormsbee and his work have been featured in many popular magazine, radio, podcast, and television outlets, including *The Washington Post*, *Men's Health*, *Shape*, *Philly.com*, and *O, The Oprah Magazine*. ∎

Table of Contents

INTRODUCTION
Professor Biography i
Course Scope 1

LECTURE GUIDES

LECTURE 1
Body Composition: Managing Our Expectations 3

LECTURE 2
A Healthier Way to Measure Body Composition. 11

LECTURE 3
How Food Is Digested and Absorbed. 20

LECTURE 4
Nutritional Needs and Cellular Function. 28

LECTURE 5
Bioenergetics: Converting Food to Energy. 37

LECTURE 6
Carbohydrates: Composition, Storage, and Use. 44

LECTURE 7
Fat: Not the Nutritional Bad Guy. 52

LECTURE 8
Protein's Critical Role in Body Composition 60

LECTURE 9
High-Protein Diets and Anabolic Resistance. 69

LECTURE 10
Critical Micronutrients and Water 78

LECTURE 11
Food Labeling and Nutritional Choices. 87

LECTURE 12
Nutrient Timing and Frequency. 95

LECTURE 13
Nighttime Eating 102

LECTURE 14
Evaluating Dietary Supplements 110

LECTURE 15
Energy Balance and Weight Control 119

LECTURE 16
The Caloric Cost of Exercise 127

LECTURE 17
Exercise for Fat Loss 134

LECTURE 18
Exercise for Healthy Muscle Mass 142

LECTURE 19
Hormones and Body Composition 149

LECTURE 20
Novel Ways to Change Body Composition. 157

LECTURE 21
Nutrition and Exercise: Special Needs 166

LECTURE 22
Set-Point Theory and the Last Five Pounds. 173

LECTURE 23
Choosing Your Nutrition Plan 181

LECTURE 24
Motivation to Change Your Body Composition. 190

SUPPLEMENTAL MATERIAL
Bibliography 197
Image Credits 239

Disclaimer

This series of lectures is intended to convey general health, fitness, and nutritional information and is for educational purposes only. It is not a substitute for, nor does it replace, professional medical advice, diagnosis, or treatment of health conditions. Please consult your physician or other health-care professional before beginning or changing any fitness or nutrition program to make sure that it is appropriate for your needs. If you have any concerns or questions about your health, you should always consult a physician or other health-care professional. Do not disregard, avoid, or delay obtaining medical or health-related advice from your health-care professional because of something you may have seen or heard in these lectures. Current health and fitness research may exist that could affect the educational information provided in these lectures, and advice found herein may not be based on the most recent findings or developments. Therefore, the use of any information provided in these lectures is solely at your own risk. By continuing with the programs, exercises, advice, information, or diets discussed in these lectures, you recognize that there are risks of injury or illness that can occur because of your use of the aforementioned information, and you expressly assume such risks and waive, relinquish, and release any claim that you may have against The Teaching Company as a result of any future physical injury or illness incurred in connection with, or as a result of, use or misuse of the programs, exercises, advice, diets, and/or information discussed in these lectures. The opinions and positions provided in these lectures reflect the opinions and positions of the relevant lecturer and do not necessarily reflect the opinions or positions of The Teaching Company or its affiliates.

The Teaching Company expressly DISCLAIMS LIABILITY for any DIRECT, INDIRECT, INCIDENTAL, SPECIAL, OR CONSEQUENTIAL DAMAGES OR LOST PROFITS that result directly or indirectly from the use of these lectures. In states that do not allow some or all of the above limitations of liability, liability shall be limited to the greatest extent allowed by law.

Acknowledgments

Sam Kramer

Brittan Allman

Katie Gorman

Stacy Cappadona

Amber Kinsey

Palmer Johnson

Chris Bach

Morgan Clift

Beth Miller

Changing Body Composition through Diet and Exercise

Scope

Improving body composition by losing body fat and optimizing lean muscle mass is not about vanity—it's about health. It's not about how quickly you can lose weight or how small you can become. It's about how to become stronger and healthier while decreasing your body fat and increasing your muscle mass. It's about changing your body composition through diet and exercise in a safe way that supports you holistically and helps you achieve optimal health and performance. This course is about the science of nutrition and exercise that can lead to lasting changes in body composition.

In the first section of the course, you will learn why body weight is not the best way to determine your health status and why understanding more about exactly how much body fat you have and how much muscle mass you have is the key to improved health and performance. You will discover what happens to food from the moment it enters your mouth—where it goes and how it supports your cellular functions. You will learn about what carbohydrates, fats, and proteins are and how they are broken down in your body to provide energy for everything you do. You will also discover that as you age, your nutrition needs change.

The next part of the course explores how to evaluate a nutrition label, and you'll discover that the calories from a bag of chips are entirely different from the same number of calories from a piece of fruit or lean meat. You'll consider how not only your food choices, but also when you eat and how frequently you eat might influence how you feel, look, and perform day to day in your normal life and also while you exercise. You'll also uncover myths and facts about dietary supplements that are designed to help you lose body fat or gain muscle mass all within the context of energy balance and weight control.

The third segment of the course examines the caloric cost of exercise, and you'll learn some simple strategies that help increase your activity level. You will discover why certain types of exercise might be most beneficial for losing body fat or gaining muscle mass. This section allows you to draw conclusions for the most optimal way for you to incorporate various types of exercise into your life to meet your goals. You'll also discover why weight training is good for everyone and won't just make you big and bulky. You will also explore certain hormones and the influence they have on your body composition.

The final lectures will use science to dispel myths about unrealistic methods that are marketed to improve body composition and provide evidence for what really works. You'll also discover the best practices for handling travel, boredom, and a busy schedule while keeping your nutrition and workout plan consistent. You will learn why improvements in body composition tend to plateau and how the set point influences your outcomes. You'll discover the science behind popular diets and how to build sustainable habits for successful loss of body fat and gain in muscle mass.

By the end of this course, you will learn to avoid the quick-fix mentality and find simple strategies to keep discipline, hard work, and fun in your plan to improve body composition. You will appreciate the complexity of the human body and understand why smart nutrition and purposeful exercise are both critical for improving body composition, health, and performance.

Body Composition: Managing Our Expectations

This course is about the science of nutrition and exercise that can lead to changes in body composition. The goal of the course is to provide you with the tools to make the decisions that you want to make, when you want to make them, to produce lasting results, not necessarily fast results. This course will provide you with all of the information you need to make big or small changes to live a fit life. The field of nutrient metabolism, exercise physiology, body composition, and performance—also known as performance nutrition—involves studying how energy is derived from foods and how this energy fuels exercise and human movement.

Body Composition

- What is body composition, and why should it be used as your indicator of health instead of body weight? We all get crazy about body weight when what we should be talking about instead is how much muscle and how much fat we have. A two-pound fat loss and a two-pound gain in muscle would improve your body composition, health, and functionality, but it would not change your body weight.

- Body mass index (BMI), which is your weight in kilograms divided by your height in meters squared, is useful in some situations but not others. The way you hold your weight—how much fat and how much muscle you have—contributes a lot to how you look, feel, and perform (in the context of the real world—in your job, with your family, and with your general energy and enthusiasm for life—not simply on an athletic field).

- The nutrition that feeds your body and fuels the physical activity that can change your body composition is also a major component of the

3

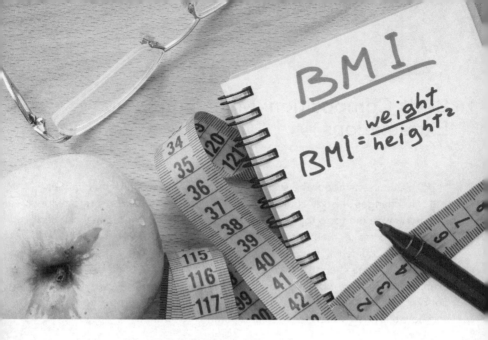

science of body composition. Nutrition is directly linked to your health and well-being. It influences your body composition and your energy levels for work, play, and exercise.

Energy Balance

- A lot of controversy surrounds the topic of energy balance. Energy balance is the balance of the calories you take in from foods and beverages (energy intake) with the calories that you expend (energy output) for all of your biological processes necessary to live, such as breathing and thinking, plus the calories you expend from walking around and from exercise.

- To alter body composition, to lose fat (for example), you want an energy deficit. Just burn more than you take in. But if it were that easy, maybe we wouldn't have the obesity epidemic that we have today.

- The quality of our calories has as much of an impact on our body composition and overall health as the total number of calories that we eat daily. Your body needs certain foods. In fact, you should probably eat more protein in your diet. Your body works harder to digest and absorb protein than it does carbohydrates and fats. This is probably why eating protein gives you the largest increase in metabolism when you eat it.

■ A number of research studies have been designed to measure metabolism after a meal containing protein versus fat versus carbohydrates, and the majority of these indicate that the greatest impact on increasing metabolism comes after eating protein. Some foods come with a little bit of a metabolic advantage, and this can have an impact on goals you're setting for changing body composition.

■ Twenty years ago, we were served smaller portion sizes. The National Institutes of Health tells us that a bagel 20 years ago was typically around 3 inches in diameter and 140 calories. Today, a bagel is typically 6 inches in diameter and contains nearly 350 calories—more than twice as many calories as just 20 years ago.

■ You don't have to begin counting calories, because that takes a lot of time and is not fun. Getting bogged down with the numbers complicates it all and can get you fixated on the wrong kinds of details. Instead, try using your hands as a way to gauge how much you should eat.

■ For example, most women can go with one palm-sized portion of lean protein to meet their needs at a particular meal. Men, who typically have bigger and thicker hands, can go with two palm-sized portions of lean protein. You simply adjust this based on your goals and the food you are eating. Carbohydrates, for example, could be a fist-sized portion of vegetables or rice.

■ Learning to pay attention to what you eat and how you feel will help you achieve your optimal body composition and lead to improved health and performance. When you eat, just eat. If you're distracted while you eat— rushed, or stressed, or not paying attention—you are more likely to eat more than your body really wants or needs. Most of the time, the simple practice of eating just enough becomes overcomplicated by massive amounts of media propaganda, misinformation, or family habits.

Exercise

- How much exercise do you need to do, and how often do you need to do it? What exercise or activity works best if you want to gain muscle mass, and what works best if you want to lose fat?

- Data shows that we lose about 5 percent of our muscle mass per decade. Over the span of 50 years, you could lose as much as 25 percent of your muscle mass. That's not something we want. It can make you weak and frail and lower your metabolism a lot, too.

- But the fact is that the overall decrease in your metabolism is only one to three percent during the aging process, which really doesn't amount to much—and you can easily offset this with the nutrition and exercise strategies that you'll learn throughout this course.

- Many people think that being sedentary is easier than being active. Screen time—the time that people watch television, use the Internet, play video games, or look at their phones—is increasing every year. This is likely a big problem because during these activities, we're usually not moving.

- In a national sample of girls and boys, it was found that those who watched less than two hours of television per day had about a 10 percent chance of becoming obese, but those who watched more than five hours per day had close to a 30 percent chance of becoming obese.

- For adults, this is also an issue—typically from too much sitting and sedentary time during the day. In fact, a number of research studies link daily sitting time to a number of health concerns, including risk of obesity, cardiovascular disease, and cancer.

- The obvious answer is to exercise. Unfortunately, planned exercise and unplanned activity typically slow down as we age and make it likely for us to gain weight and fat. You need to make a real effort to stop this reduction in metabolism and work for your optimal body composition.

■ Having the body composition of your dreams is certainly a great goal, but keep in mind that just being active is extremely helpful for improving your health. The good news is that following even the most basic of recommendations brings many benefits.

■ In fact, just a 5 to 10 percent loss in total body weight will improve your blood pressure, cholesterol, and sugar levels. And even if you're still in the "overweight" or "obese" range, this modest weight loss can decrease your risk factors for chronic diseases related to obesity.

■ A major point of information about body composition that most people don't know is that if you are trying to lose weight, you should be lifting weights. This might go against what you've always been told, but long and slow aerobic exercise is no longer the recommended way to lose fat. While it is part of the plan, many other types of exercise are needed if you really want a fighting chance to lose fat but keep or add muscle mass.

■ Particularly when trying to lose weight, it's important to lift weights so that your muscle mass has the best chance of staying around and your metabolism stays as high as possible.

■ Quick changes in body composition should not be expected. Instead, look for changes to come over a period of time, after you've dialed in a nourishing eating plan based on quality foods and a consistent and effective exercise regimen.

Nutrition

■ Overall, the health benefits of exercise and eating right are clear. If a pill existed with even half of the same benefits, there's no doubt that it would be the best seller.

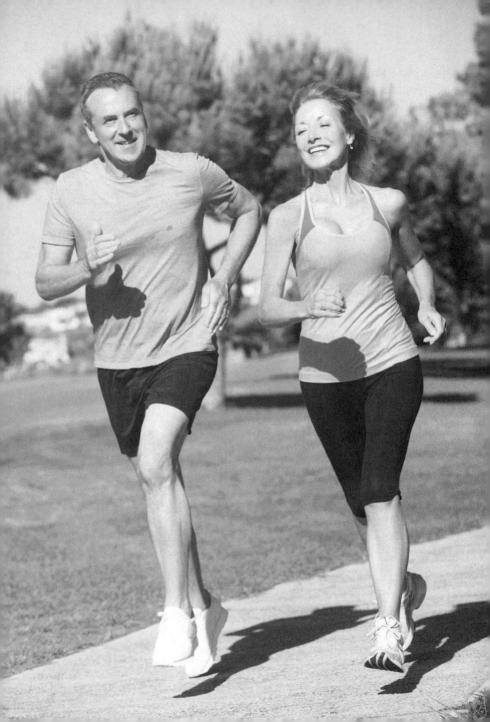

- Even if you are overweight or obese, simply being physically active can ward off metabolic disease and keep you healthy. Health is not always about weight. Of course, they are related, but the key for your health is that you exercise and work on ways to improve how you eat.

- However, simply exercising more and eating less is not the key for improving body composition. We've been preaching this for a long time, but it doesn't work very well. The science of healthy body composition is not weight loss science; it's the science of a healthy balance of fat and muscle mass and how we can achieve that.

- Choosing both quality exercise and quality foods is the way to make lasting improvements. And weight loss might be a consequence of changing eating and exercise habits, but it is not the goal.

- It's also important to keep in mind that things like your genetics, your environment, and even chemical pollutants are factors that might contribute to gaining fat. But even though our ability to alter our body composition depends on many things, the take-home message is that exercise and quality nutrition do a body good.

- In fact, exercise and nutrition must be combined for a healthy body composition. You can make it pretty far with one or the other, but healthy does not just mean "not overweight."

- Your journey to better health is not about a quick fix; it's about a lifestyle change that works for you. It's not about how quickly you can lose weight or how small you can become. It's about how to become stronger and healthier while lowering your body fat and increasing your muscle mass. It's about changing your body composition through diet and exercise in a safe way that supports you holistically and helps you achieve more day to day.

Try This

Write down the biggest hurdle you see as standing in the way of achieving your optimal body composition and health.

Questions to Consider

1. What is the easiest and most sustainable change that you think you can make for big improvements in your body composition, health, and performance?

2. What exercise or nutrition myth was busted by this lecture?

A Healthier Way to Measure Body Composition

Body weight offers no indication of how much fat versus muscle a person carries on his or her frame. This relative proportion is critical, because it is related to what the status of our overall health is, how our body moves and behaves, and how we look and feel aesthetically. How can we better quantify success with weight management? After this lecture, you will have a better, healthier idea of what's happening to your body during weight loss, which benchmarks are typically used to indicate success, and why success goes far beyond simply what the scale tells you.

Body Mass Index and Fat-Free Mass Index

- Body mass index (BMI) compares your body weight (in kilograms) to your height (in meters squared). A note of caution: Measures like BMI or body weight may be relevant only in certain situations. The usefulness of BMI is not great when considered on an individual-to-individual basis. In practice, BMI is most appropriate for large sample populations or in a clinical situation to quantify risk for a patient who is clearly overweight and overfat at the same time.

- There are four main categories of BMI.
  - Underweight: a BMI of less than 18.5.
  - Normal weight: 18.5 to 24.9.
  - Overweight: 25 to 29.
  - Obese: more than 30.

- Research has consistently shown a positive association between a high BMI and greater risk of cardiovascular, pulmonary, and metabolic disease. If you are curious about your own body mass index, calculate it or look online for a free website that can give you the information.

- The problem is that BMI only considers your body weight and body height and does not account for the proportion of muscle mass or fat mass—which is the composition of your body weight.

- For example, a typical NFL running back is very strong, has lots of lean muscle mass, and has very little body fat. Assuming that this running back is about 6 feet tall and a little more than 230 pounds (due to all of the muscle mass), his BMI would be more than 31 kg/m². According to BMI standards, this professional, healthy, lean athlete would be considered obese, even though common sense tells us otherwise.

- Body composition is different from body weight and body mass index. Body composition is the relationship between the different types of tissue that comprise your body—in other words, how much muscle and how much fat make up your body weight.

- To account for fat-free mass and not just total body weight, the fat-free mass index (FFMI) was developed. It is similar to the BMI, but it takes your fat-free mass, or muscle mass (again, in kilograms), divided by your height (in meters squared).

- This index can quantify your body composition more accurately when you know that you have extra weight that is mostly muscle. It is not always a better index, but it is a different index, and like any index will be more or less useful depending on the specific need for the information.

- While the FFMI is not used nearly as much as the BMI, a few research papers have attempted to come up with normal FFMI values for men and women. A paper from 2002 in the *International Journal of Obesity and Related Metabolic Disorders* found that the average FFMI for young women is about 15 kg/m² and for young men is 19 kg/m². These values change slightly after age 35, showing that fat mass is gained as we age, most likely due to a more sedentary lifestyle.

- These indices are important to consider because they can be helpful for knowing your health status and risk for certain kinds of disease, such as cardiovascular disease, pulmonary disease, and metabolic disease. It is well established that if you have a lot of fat deposition, particularly around your waist and belly (near your major organs), your chance of developing these types of diseases increases dramatically.

- In addition, knowing your current body composition gives you greater clarity about your starting point for an upcoming weight loss intervention. You will better be able to track your body's changes over time and have a bigger picture of "success."

MYTH
Muscle Weighs More Than Fat

This myth is just like saying that one pound of bricks weighs more than one pound of feathers: Of course, if you have one pound of each, then they both weigh one pound.

But here is the difference: Muscle has more density than fat. This is a key to understanding why two people can weigh exactly the same at the same height but look entirely different.

If you look at five pounds of fat and five pounds of muscle, they weigh exactly the same, but the amount of muscle is smaller than the same amount of fat. The muscle is about a third to a half smaller than the fat because of its increased density.

When you add muscle, you might weigh the same, but you could be an entirely different shape.

Body Fat and Muscle Mass

- In terms of body composition, your total body fat includes both essential body fat and storage body fat. Essential fat includes fat in your organs, such as the heart, liver, kidneys, intestines, muscles, and bone marrow. This type of fat is required for normal physiological functioning and differs greatly between men and women. In fact, it accounts for most of the major body fat differences between genders. Women have about 12 percent essential fat, while men have about 3 percent essential fat.

- Women have more essential fat mostly because of its biological function for reproduction. Women need extra fat stores during pregnancy. Regardless of whether a woman ever has children or not, she will most often have slightly more fat than a man.

- There is another type of fat that is also required for normal body function. It is called storage fat, which is fat stored until it can be used for energy when needed. It includes the visceral fat, or deep fat, around your organs and the fat just underneath your skin, which is called subcutaneous fat.

- Storage fat can insulate your body, helps to maintain your body temperature, and provides vital protection for your organs. The amount of storage fat is more similar between men and women—usually just 2 to 3 percent higher in women.

- Health issues arise when storage fat becomes excessive. Body fat is important for supporting daily function and health, but excess amounts will contribute to overweight and overfat conditions.

- The other component of body mass that is not comprised of fat is called fat-free mass or lean body mass. These terms are often used interchangeably; however, they are technically different. Fat-free mass is only the muscle mass that you have, while lean body mass also includes your muscle mass, bone mass, connective tissue (such as ligaments and tendons), internal organs, and any essential fat stored in these tissues.

- In practice, body composition is often described as a two-compartment model: fat mass and fat-free mass (or lean body mass). And if you know these values, it can help you avoid getting stuck in the rut of only measuring and talking about body weight. It will also give you much more information about your overall health.

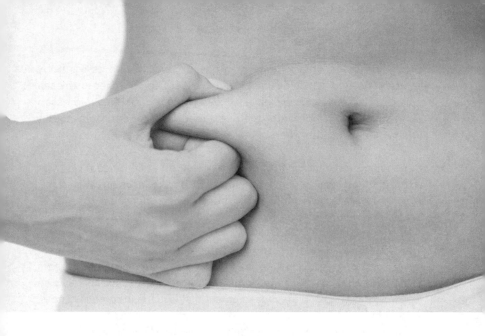

- Typically, body fat levels are broken into "optimal health" and "optimal fitness." These terms are very similar, but in general, "health" refers to the optimal level for reduced risk of disease, and "fitness" takes a step further to the optimal level for physical fitness. We should all strive for at least optimal health, and then optimal fitness.

- For women, optimal health is a body fat range of 18 to 30 percent and optimal fitness is 16 to 25 percent. For men, optimal health is 10 to 25 percent and optimal fitness is 12 to 18 percent. Consider your own goals to determine which range you should fall into. Then, the next step is to determine your current body composition.

Measuring Body Composition

- Many methods of assessing body composition exist, including direct and indirect measurements. Direct measurements include dissolution of the body and physical dissection. This means that to truly know your body composition, you will have to wait until after you have passed away and donate your body to science. This is obviously not a viable option.

■ Luckily for us, multiple indirect methods are available to assess body composition and are fairly easy to get access to. But because each method is indirect, each will have its own inherent error threshold based on the accuracy compared to the direct method. That error threshold is usually somewhere between one and four percent.

■ Depending on the modality, if you are measured at 30 percent body fat with a method that has an error threshold of plus or minus 4 percent, your "true body fat" could really be anywhere between 26 and 34 percent body fat.

■ While this is somewhat disappointing, these assessment tools are great for tracking changes over time, as long as the same machine and same technician is doing the measuring. The skill of the technician can also make big differences in the measurement that is made in some instances.

■ Some of the more expensive and laboratory-based methods include the following.
   ◆ Dual-energy X-ray absorptiometry (DEXA)
   ◆ Hydrostatic, or underwater, weighing
   ◆ Air-displacement plethysmography, or what is commonly known as the "bod pod"
   ◆ Skinfold measurements using skinfold pinches
   ◆ Bioelectrical impedance analysis using an electrical current
   ◆ Advanced clinical methods, such as computerized tomography (CT) or magnetic resonance imaging (MRI)

■ With each technique, we are able to assess body density through your body volume in water (such as with underwater weighing) or in air (such as with the bod pod), or via some sort of imaging technique, such as DEXA, CT, or MRI.

■ For most of these tests, you can either ask your local gym personnel to administer them or search for a human performance or exercise science laboratory at a local college or university.

Body Shape

■ All of these methods can only estimate your relative fat and lean components. But just how much body fat you have is not the whole picture. It turns out that where you store that fat may be more important than how much fat you have.

■ Typically, fat is stored either around your abdomen in the typical "apple shape," called android fat, or around your hips and buttocks in the typical "pear shape," called gynoid fat. Depending on where you store your fat, you can often predict your risk of future health complications.

■ The android pattern of body fat indicates a lot of fat stored around your organs, which is called visceral fat, in addition to fat also underneath your skin, which is called subcutaneous fat. This fat distribution is much

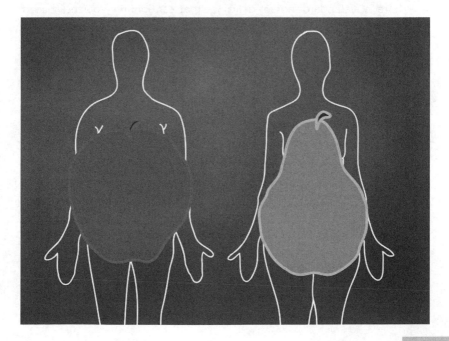

more common in men and is associated with more disease risk than the gynoid fat distributions.

- The gynoid fat deposition is typically thought of as the female pattern of weight gain. This might actually be protective against disease for women. However, after menopause, when estrogen production tapers off, women tend to shift more toward the android obesity that is associated with men.

- A measurement called waist-to-hip ratio, or waist and hip circumference, was developed to quickly and easily allow physicians to crudely estimate body composition as well as determine risk based on where fat is located. The size of your waist (smallest part of your abdomen) in relation to your hips (greatest protrusion of the buttocks) can quickly paint the picture of your fat distribution.

- There is a standardized set of values that can identify your risk based on both measurements. For example, your disease risk increases with a total waist circumference measurement of more than 35 inches (88.9 cm) for women and more than 40 inches (101.6 cm) for men. And this is for just for your waist, regardless of hip circumference.

- Similarly, a waist-to-hip ratio of greater than 0.86 for women or greater than 0.95 for men indicates an increased risk for disease. The closer to 1 or above, meaning a bigger belly than buttocks, gives you the apple shape. In both cases, improvements in body composition are recommended to avoid these associated health problems.

- Another way that body shape is often described is according to somatotype, or physique shape. The three clearly defined shapes include ectomorphs, who are naturally thin with longer limbs and small joints; mesomorphs, who are naturally muscular with broad shoulders and narrow waists; and endomorphs, who are more round and soft with thicker joints.

■ Most people can identify with one of the categories even if they are a hybrid of two groups. Just keep in mind that the type of body shape you might naturally be might be hidden or morphed by years of beating up your body with excess food or, on the other hand, lots of dedicated exercise to change your body composition.

■ Regardless, these body shapes are correlated with certain levels of fat mass and muscle mass. Knowing which category you fall into can also help you set realistic goals for body composition and performance.

Try This

Find your starting point and work with a fitness professional to have your body fat percent measured.

Questions to Consider

1. Why should you care more about body composition than body weight?

2. Why might lifting weights change your waist size but not your body weight?

How Food Is Digested and Absorbed

Every bit of the food you eat has a dramatic impact on your body composition, health, and how you feel. The bulk of this lecture will focus on the details of digestion and absorption. It will also touch on how the aging process can interfere with normal digestion absorption—and how that can affect body composition. You'll also learn about nutrient partitioning, which is the manipulation of both nutrient content and nutrient timing of your diet for specific physiological reasons.

Digestion and Absorption

- How does the food you eat enter into your body for storage as glycogen (stored carbohydrate), fat, or protein? Many processes must happen inside your body to prepare food for use or storage.

- Before the food you eat can be used for energy, it needs to be broken down inside the body into individual nutrients. This is digestion. Following digestion, the body must take up, or absorb, the individual nutrients to either use them or store them for later. This is called absorption.

- Foods and beverages provide your body with nutrients that it needs to sustain itself. The nutrients for our body are split into two main categories: macronutrients and micronutrients.

- Macronutrients, consisting of carbohydrates, fats, and proteins, are used by your body's cells to create energy. Micronutrients—vitamins, minerals, and water—do not provide calories, or energy, but they are required for many physiological processes in the body, including digestion and absorption.

- Once you take a bite of food, the first section of the gastrointestinal (GI) tract that it hits is the mouth. The food then travels down the esophagus and enters the stomach to be chemically and mechanically broken down into smaller fragments.

- After the stomach, these food fragments enter the small intestine, followed by the large intestine. Whatever nutrients and materials the body does not use up until this point are excreted through the rectum and anal canal.

- Along the route, your pancreas, gallbladder, and liver all help digest and absorb the food by producing various enzymes (specialty proteins that help reactions occur) and enzyme solutions that help break down and transport foods.

- Almost all nutrients within the food you eat must be digested before they are absorbed. Various physical and chemical activities from the mouth, stomach, pancreas, and small intestine are responsible for digestion.

- Once all of the nutrients are broken down into their simplest forms, they are then taken up into the cells of the GI tract to be transported throughout the entire body. This process is known as absorption.

- Most of the carbohydrates, fats, and proteins that you consume are generally absorbed within 30 minutes after reaching the small intestines. Any intestinal material that is not absorbed by the time it reaches the end of the last portion of the small intestine passes through something called the ileocecal valve and then into the large intestine.

- Overall, it can take anywhere from 12 to 70 hours for food remnants to pass all the way through the colon, and waste products are eventually excreted as fecal matter through the anal canal.

- Your body composition overall is highly influenced by the digestion and absorption of nutrients from the food you eat.

Carbohydrates

- Through digestion, more complex carbohydrates are eventually broken down into individual units, known as monosaccharides. The three monosaccharides are glucose, galactose, and fructose, with the most common being glucose.

- Most nutrients are absorbed somewhere along the length of the small intestine, through the brush border—where all of the intestinal digestive enzymes are produced and stored—into the intestinal cells. Carbohydrates are absorbed very efficiently and are usually cleared out of the small intestine more quickly than fats or proteins.

- Glucose is absorbed into the intestinal cells by a protein complex called the sodium-glucose transporter. This is an "active" process, meaning that energy, or adenosine triphosphate (ATP), is required to make this happen.

- After glucose is absorbed into the intestinal cell, it is then transported out of the cell and into the bloodstream. Some of the glucose simply diffuses into the blood, but a carrier protein transports much of the glucose from the intestinal cell into the blood.

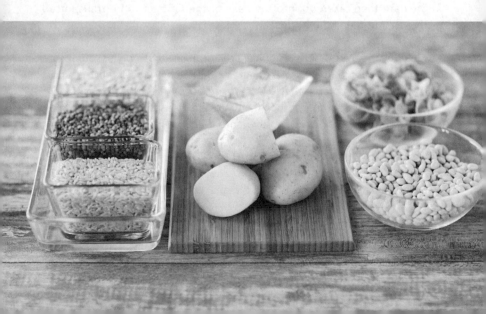

- Once glucose enters the blood, it goes directly to the liver. This is called portal circulation. The liver is the main site of glucose metabolism, so it gets first choice on what to do with the incoming glucose: use it, store it, or let it move on.

- Any glucose that is not metabolized and used in the liver passes through to systemic, or whole-body, circulation. From here, glucose travels to various other tissues, where it can be taken up through a facilitated transport process, using other transport proteins before it is used within that tissue.

Fat

- Digestion of fat begins in the mouth by the action of an enzyme called lingual lipase. Only very small amounts are broken down in the stomach. The bulk of triglyceride (or fat) digestion occurs in the small intestine.

- Before fats are broken into their component parts, they must first be emulsified by bile. Bile is produced in the liver but stored in the gallbladder.

- Once fat is present in the small intestine, a hormone called cholecystokinin (CCK) is secreted, and then bile is released through the bile ducts into the small intestine, and the emulsification process begins.

- Once emulsified, pancreatic lipase acts on the fats and further breaks them into smaller units that can be absorbed and transported for use.

- Unlike carbohydrates, fats are a little tricky when it comes to their absorption and transportation. They are naturally insoluble in water. Because of this, they cannot move through the brush border or the blood as individual lipid units.

- To solve this problem, broken-down fat particles mix with bile salts and form a water-soluble substance called a micelle, which then interacts at the brush border of the small intestine. Fat particles move out of the micelle and into the intestinal cell, and the water-soluble bile salts continue down through the small intestine until they are reabsorbed and sent back to the liver.

- After the broken-down fat particles—which include free fatty acids, monoglycerides, and some cholesterol and phospholipid particles—are in the intestinal cell, they actually combine back together to their larger original triglyceride form. Then, they are transported.

- Fats are not only broken down differently than carbohydrates; they also travel differently. Fats must travel through the lymph system instead of the blood. The lymphatic system is a network of vessels that transports nutrients to the cells and collects cell waste products.

- In a slow process, fats move out into the lymphatic vessels and eventually into the blood, where they freely travel to tissues to deliver the fats for use or storage. Some fat will be used by your muscle cells to produce energy, and some will be deposited into your fat cells.

- There are many things that affect how fats are used and stored, including when you last ate, what your overall calorie intake for the day and exercise habits are, and how physically fit you are.

- Because the transportation process for fats is relatively slow, it could take anywhere from 30 minutes to 3 hours after you eat a high-fat meal for your blood lipids to reach the highest level. About 5 to 6 hours after the meal, however, the fats will have been delivered to the designated tissues, and your blood levels should return to normal.

Protein

- The structure of protein is very complex. The reason that digestion of protein makes more demands on the body's metabolism is because of the complexity of protein.

■ Proteins stay fully intact until they get to your stomach. Large proteins are broken down into individual amino acids in the stomach by very acidic stomach juice. Proteins that are still intact after leaving the stomach are broken down further in the top portion of the small intestine. The end products of protein digestion are free amino acids, which are absorbed into the intestinal cell.

■ Proteins are absorbed in a process more similar to carbohydrates than fats. This process occurs along the entire small intestine.

■ Amino acids, just like glucose, require a sodium-dependent carrier to get into the intestinal cells. There are several uses for particular amino acids within the intestinal cell. However, amino acids that are not used within the intestinal cells themselves are transported out of the cells into the blood and make their first stop at the liver.

■ About 50 to 65 percent of all ingested amino acids are metabolized in the liver. The rest of the amino acids are used in other tissues, particularly the skeletal muscles, kidneys, and brain.

Micronutrients

■ Macronutrients provide the body with energy. Micronutrients, on the other hand, do not provide energy. Despite this, micronutrients are vital to make all of the digestive processes occur, along with hundreds of other reactions and processes within the body.

■ Water-soluble vitamins—vitamin C and all B-complex vitamins—are absorbed into and transported through the blood. With the exception of vitamin B_{12}, water-soluble vitamins are not stored in the body for long periods of time. They are either used fairly quickly in the body or are excreted in the urine, so we need to get them daily from the food we eat.

■ Fat-soluble vitamins—vitamins A, D, E, and K—are absorbed and transported much like fats. Unlike water-soluble vitamins, excess fat-soluble vitamins can be stored in the body for a decent amount of time. For this reason, fat-soluble vitamins deficiencies are much less common than water-soluble vitamin deficiencies.

Anorexia of Aging

- For the most part, the GI tract of a healthy individual works like a well-oiled machine. Along with the digestive system itself, the endocrine and nervous systems play a major role in regulating digestion, absorption, and transportation of nutrients.

- Unfortunately, as people start to age, some functions of these systems begin to slow down. The main cause for these changes is the degeneration of the enteric nervous system, which is the nervous system of the GI tract. This can lead to serious GI complications.

- Along with biological and nervous system complications, elderly individuals might experience what has come to be known as "anorexia of aging." This refers to a physiological age-related reduction in appetite and energy intake, which leads to significant weight loss and muscle wasting.

- Basically, as you age, there might come a time when you just don't feel hungry very often. While this might lead to weight loss, this is not a good thing; oftentimes muscle mass is lost, too. Ultimately, low muscle mass prevents mobility.

- Your best bet to avoid or slow this age-related reduction in appetite is to simply make sure that you are leading a healthy lifestyle. See your doctor regularly, exercise, and nourish yourself with foods that contribute to your health.

Nutrient Partitioning

- Nutrient partitioning is the term used to describe how the food you eat is stored or partitioned into a specific storage area, such as muscle or fat. At the most basic level, the more of one type of food you eat—carbohydrates, fats, or protein—the more of that fuel you will burn for energy.

■ Exercise is the most important and powerful tool to help you use the foods you eat to improve body composition. If you are active, you will tend to use the foods you eat to power exercise. But if you are sedentary, your body will tend to partition the foods you eat to being stored as fat, instead of being used and stored for a healthy purpose.

Try This

Pay attention to the foods you eat and how they make you feel and perform.

Questions to Consider

1. Why is nutrient digestion and absorption important to body composition?

2. What is the biggest determinant of nutrient partitioning?

Nutritional Needs and Cellular Function

I
t is very easy to associate the food you eat with external, appearance-driven end points like body weight. But it's important to understand how the food you eat affects you on the inside, because your internal functioning directly influences how you feel, how you look, and your overall health. The nutrients you eat are an ingrained part of every cell and tissue that makes you what you are and who you are. In this lecture, you will learn which nutrients are needed to keep your cells healthy and what these nutrients actually do inside your body.

Cells in the Human Body

- The cell is the smallest structural and functional unit of any organism. It is what every living being is made out of.

- Our cells vary immensely in size, function, and chemical makeup. Each cell is a minute version of a human life. Each cell in our body must move, grow, consume food, excrete waste products, react to the environment it lives in, and reproduce.

- Cells in the human body are constantly communicating to make the entire organism function. They communicate in response to your environment, what you touch, and how you move.

- Cells bond together to make tissues; tissues make up our organs; our organs make up all of our organ systems; and our organ systems combine to make up the organism, which, in this case, is our body.

- If your cells are not healthy, then they will not work properly. If the cells don't work properly, then the tissues won't work properly. If tissues aren't working, then the systems will begin to fail. Eventually, you will most likely experience increased fatigue, decreased physical capacity, improper nutrient use, and partitioning, which might ultimately lead to poor body composition as well as serious health consequences.

■ By keeping your cells healthy and fed with the proper nutrients, you are keeping your whole self healthy.

■ The average adult human body is made up of about 30 trillion cells. When the old cells become damaged, new ones are made to replace them. The nutrients we get from our food are used to make these new cells. This is the main reason why nutrition plays such a major role in cellular health and, therefore, in overall optimal functioning.

■ Also, certain nutrients from the food we eat can protect cells from early damage and provide the cells with the fuel needed to produce energy for our bodies.

Cell Components

■ The outermost component of the cell is the cell membrane. It is the boundary that separates the internal components of the cell from the outside environment. It keeps all of the cellular contents safe so that they can function properly without being damaged.

■ The cell membrane is referred to as "semipermeable," meaning that it has the ability to filter out important nutrients from damaging waste products. The membrane allows various nutrients to pass through the wall and sends the wastes out to be removed from the body. The permeability of this membrane also allows the cells to communicate clearly with one another.

■ All of the dietary macronutrients—carbohydrates, fats, and proteins—are found in the cell membrane. The most abundant form of fat found in the cell membrane is the phospholipids, which have a hydrophobic, or water-fearing, tail and a hydrophilic, or water-loving, head. This love-hate relationship with water is what gives the membrane its unique structure and stability.

- Another type of fat-related compound found in the cell membrane is cholesterol. The cholesterol improves the mechanical stability of the membrane and helps regulate the fluidity.

- The second major nutrient found in the cell membrane is protein. Proteins play a small role in forming the structure of the membrane, but they mostly contribute to the membrane functions. They direct proper operation within each individual cell and also the healthy functioning of your entire body.

- Lastly, carbohydrates are also found in the cell membrane, but in smaller amounts compared to fats and proteins. Carbohydrates contribute to membrane structure and are present in the form of glycoproteins and glycolipids, which are protein and lipid molecules that have a glucose or sugar residue attached. These molecules also typically function to support cellular signaling.

- The next important cellular structure that is essentially built from our foods is the nucleus. The nucleus is the largest organelle, or specialized structure, within the cell, and it contains the cell's DNA.

- The nuclear envelope surrounds the nucleus. This two-layer membrane is composed primarily of lipids and proteins. It also contains minerals that are needed for activities within the nucleus.

- The nucleus can be referred to as your "genetic storehouse" because it contains all of your personal information within its nuclear membrane walls in the DNA.

- DNA is the blueprint for every one of the body's proteins. The proteins that make up your tissues, organs, chemical messengers, and more originate from the coding of DNA and the quality of food that we eat.

- For this reason, it is vital that the nucleus has a solid structure to keep the DNA safe from damage that occurs from normal metabolic and oxidative stresses and aging. Nutrition also plays an important role in protecting your DNA.

- Another cellular structure is the mitochondria. Known as the "powerhouse" of the cell, the mitochondria are responsible for energy production. All of the nutrients from your food are turned into energy within the microscopic mitochondria of your cells.

- Just like the cell membrane and nuclear membrane, the mitochondrial membrane is made up of fats and proteins. The mitochondrial membrane has an inner and outer membrane, both of which play important roles in energy processes. The mitochondria also use many micronutrients to assist with producing energy.

- The structural and functional integrity of the mitochondrial membrane is critical to your health. If the mitochondria structure and/or function is compromised, energy production from that cell will be compromised. This mitochondrial dysfunction can contribute to several chronic diseases, including diabetes, heart disease, and Parkinson's disease.

Omegas

- Unsaturated fats are necessary for strong cell membranes. The membrane is semipermeable thanks to the fluid structure of the fats. However, saturated and trans fats are much more rigid than unsaturated fats. They don't function the same way as the unsaturated fats, and they cause membranes to be much more rigid than what is optimal, potentially limiting the functionality of cells.

- Diets that are too high in one type of fat—for example, trans fats— might lead to rigid and brittle cell membranes that cannot communicate as well as if they were composed of a better mix of fat types. In general, diets high in unsaturated fats will promote healthy cell membranes.

- Two categories of unsaturated fats to take particular note of are omega-6 fatty acids and omega-3 fatty acids.

- Omega-6 fatty acids are highly concentrated in walnuts, almonds, and various types of vegetable oils, including corn, soybean, safflower, cottonseed, sunflower seed, and peanut oil.

- Rich sources of omega-3 fatty acids include fatty fish, such as salmon, tuna, cod, and trout. Some seeds and nuts also contain omega-3 fatty acids, such as flaxseed, but to a much lower extent.

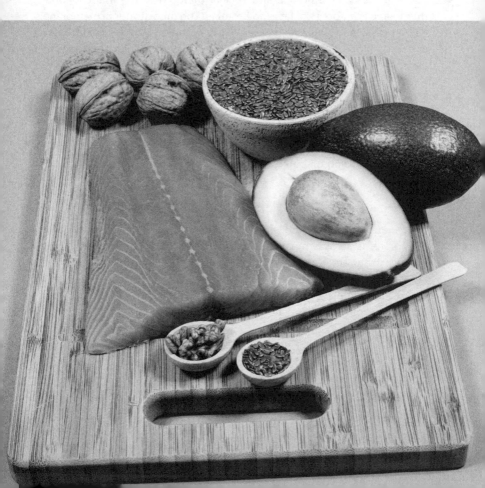

■ Both omega-6 and omega-3 fatty acids are essential for good health; however, they both play very different roles. Omega-3 fatty acids have an anti-inflammatory effect in the body, whereas omega-6 fatty acids have a pro-inflammatory effect.

■ While some amount of inflammation can help protect the body from infection and injury, too much inflammation can lead to heart disease, metabolic syndrome, diabetes, Alzheimer's disease, arthritis, and many different types of cancer. As opposed to omega-6 fatty acids, omega-3 fatty acids are known to lower the risk of these diseases by decreasing the amount of inflammation within the body.

■ Other nutrients required to maintain healthy cell membranes include high-quality proteins, fat-soluble vitamins (vitamins A, D, E, and K), and vitamin C. Whole grains, vegetables, fruits, and lean poultry and fish will provide you with all of these nutrients and will keep your cell membranes in top shape.

■ Because the cell nucleus and your DNA are also made up of nutrients, the quality of food you eat can greatly impact their structure and function as well. Unfortunately, despite the barrier provided by the nucleus, DNA can be damaged from any excess potentially harmful substances (often called toxins) circulating around in the body.

■ Damage to DNA can also occur from reactive oxygen species or excessive oxidative stress, which can be produced as by-products from the energy we produce from food or even from excessive exercise.

■ If reactive oxygen species make their way into the nuclear membrane, they can potentially alter normal DNA functioning. If this occurs, the proteins that the particular DNA strand produced will no longer be available to your body. This will lead to poor functioning in your body and could lead to various disease states.

- One way to protect this from happening is by eating quality sources of polyunsaturated fats. You can focus on getting these fats from sources like fatty fish, flaxseeds, walnuts, and even soybeans.

- Other nutrients that are needed to protect DNA include high-quality protein, antioxidants, and vitamins. The easiest way to get these nutrients into your diet is to consume foods like lean meat, eggs, dairy, colorful vegetables, whole grains, and fruits.

B Vitamins, Iron, Sulfur

- The mitochondria can use the nutrients we eat and turn them into energy for everything we do. However, not all foods are created equal when it comes to efficiency of energy production.

- Most of the energy that the mitochondria produce comes from fats and glucose (carbohydrate) either stored in your body or from your diet. This energy ultimately ends up in the form of adenosine triphosphate (ATP).

- The process of making ATP from our foods is very complex. The obvious nutrients that are needed for these processes to occur are the energy-yielding macronutrients: carbohydrates, fats, and proteins. However, essential nutrients that are often overlooked when talking about energy production are the B vitamins, iron, and sulfur.

- The B vitamins work to transfer electrons through the electron transport chain, which produces a massive amount of ATP in your mitochondria. Iron and sulfur are important components of the protein structures within the major energy-producing systems of your cells and are used to simply transport oxygen around your body.

- If iron and sulfur are not available from the diet to the mitochondria, energy production will suffer. Just as with the cell membranes and the nuclear membranes, nutritional support for healthy mitochondria function comes from eating foods with a lot of nutrients that are minimally processed. Things like green leafy vegetables, complex carbohydrates, and lean proteins are a great start.

Exercise Levels

- Some factors that have nothing to do with food can also impact our cellular health and function. For example, excessive exercise can actually cause some damage. Exercise naturally increases the production of free radicals, which are molecules that have an unpaired electron in their outer shell. The missing electron in these molecules causes them to be unstable and highly reactive.

- To regain stability, the free radical molecule works to steal electrons from healthy cells in your body. When this happens, the free radical leaves a healthy cell damaged and unable to perform its usual functions.

- This free radical damage does not stop with one cell. Once one free radical attack occurs, it sets off a domino effect. The newly damaged cells move on to other healthy cells as they attempt to become neutral again. Excessive free radical damage has been associated with accelerated aging, cancer, diabetes, and coronary artery disease.

- Luckily, our bodies have the ability to fight free radical attacks by forming three natural antioxidants: glutathione, catalase, and superoxide dismutase. These substances donate extra electrons to free radicals and prevent them from damaging healthy cells.

- The major problem with exercise occurs when it is too extreme, causing the production of free radicals to exceed the body's ability to produce antioxidants. This does not mean that you should shy away from all intense exercise, however, because your diet can help ward off this exercise-induced oxidative stress—a diet that includes lots of fruits and vegetables that are full of antioxidants.

- Being still and sedentary can also have a negative impact on cellular health and integrity. Sedentary lifestyles are associated with increased cardiovascular disease, atherosclerosis, overweight/obesity, diabetes, accelerated aging, and more. Oxidative stress plays a major role in these dysfunctions. Sedentary lifestyles can lead to increased oxidative stress and vascular dysfunction.

■ Leading a physically active life (but not excessively active or sedentary) will help keep our cells healthy, happy, and functioning to the best of their ability.

Try This

Try eating more omega-3 fatty acids to decrease your ratio of omega-6 to omega-3 fatty acids.

Questions to Consider

1. What is really meant by "you are what you eat"?

2. Provide an example for where specific foods you eat are used for your cellular functioning.

Bioenergetics: Converting Food to Energy

I n this lecture, you will learn how we produce energy from the food we eat and which food choices might be best based on your activity level. Knowing how to use your energy systems to your advantage is a huge asset when wanting to change your body composition. After digesting and absorbing the food you eat, it is amazing how it is used to provide energy for everything you want to do, including changing your body composition.

Bioenergetics and Metabolism

- Bioenergetics is the process of converting the components of the foods we eat—such as carbohydrates, fats, and proteins—into a usable form of energy. Bioenergetics relates directly to your overall metabolism, which is the sum of all energy transformations that occur in your body.

- We produce energy by converting the food we eat into adenosine triphosphate (ATP), which is often called the "energy currency" of the body because in a sense we "pay" for all of our biological actions with ATP.

- To release the energy from ATP, it is broken apart in a process called hydrolysis, using an enzyme called ATPase. ATP is broken apart into smaller components to produce adenosine diphosphate (ADP), a single phosphate, and energy.

- Food is eaten and eventually converted to energy (ATP), carbon dioxide, and water. And the ATP is used to produce work for all of your metabolic needs and daily activities. Heat is also produced in the process of making energy.

- Essentially, you simply changed the chemical composition of the food you eat into other forms of useable energy and heat. This follows the first law of thermodynamics, which states that energy is neither created nor destroyed, but only changed in form.

- ATP is the stored chemical energy that links the energy-producing and energy-requiring functions within all cells. This energy fuels all forms of biological work, such as digestion of food and muscle contractions.

Making and Replacing Stores of ATP

- We have three energy systems that make and replace our stores of ATP for us. In all three systems, a phosphate group is added to an adenosine diphosphate (ADP) molecule in a process called phosphorylation to create adenosine triphosphate (ATP). That phosphate is added to ADP and then stored as ATP until the energy from ATP is needed for activities, such as exercising.

- Each energy system has a specific role and works at the highest rate based on how hard or intensely you are working. Each system has a different way of providing ATP, but they are used on a continuum and overlap quite a bit.

- In addition, certain parts of each of the three energy systems can also work to provide ATP in the other two energy systems. In this way, you get the most ATP out of whatever you are doing and whatever fuel source—carbohydrates, fats, or proteins—you are using to provide energy.

- By understanding these energy systems, you will gain the ability to decide what to eat, or what certain nutrients may be best to support whatever you are doing. This allows you to better understand how to eat what you can use best for energy production, limit storing excess body fat, and improve success in fat loss.

- The three energy-producing systems are the creatine phosphate system, the glycolytic system, and the oxidative system. All of these systems are at work for us to provide energy, but one system is typically used more than the others during different exercise and rest scenarios.

■ The creatine phosphate system works hardest for us during maximal-intensity exercise. In this system, you will create ATP by first combining a phosphate with stored creatine, which is a combination of amino acids, to form creatine phosphate. Then, the enzyme creatine kinase breaks off the phosphate from creatine phosphate and allows it to combine with ADP. This forms more ATP and free creatine.

■ This process is anaerobic, meaning that it occurs without oxygen. This does not mean that you aren't taking in oxygen by breathing; it just means that ATP can be produced without the presence of oxygen in the cells.

■ The creatine phosphate energy system works quickly but does not last for long; about 30 seconds is all you'll get (depending on your fitness level), but it is the most rapid method to regenerate ATP.

■ The second energy system is the glycolytic system, also called anaerobic glycolysis, which relies on carbohydrates as a fuel source to make energy. The glycolytic system lasts longer than the creatine phosphate system—but probably not more than about two minutes while you are working hard. Once again, you produce ATP without the need for oxygen in your cells.

■ Glycolysis is the breakdown of carbohydrates or glucose to make ATP. Glucose is in any type of carbohydrate that you eat or drink, such as a sports drink or piece of bread. Once the glucose is in your blood, you need to get it into your cells to break it down to either make ATP or store it as glycogen for later use.

■ You can use stored glycogen or the glucose from food that you've recently eaten to make ATP. In both cases, you first need to get the glucose into your cells. There is an elaborate system of proteins called GLUT transporters that assist with this. The glycolytic energy system is one you rely on a lot during any kind of physical activity.

- The third energy system is the oxidative system, which relies on carbohydrates, fats, and in some cases protein to provide ATP. The oxidative system is the long and slow system, which kicks in after about 90 seconds to 2 minutes of activity and can last almost indefinitely—as long as the intensity of activity is low to moderate. It's aerobic, unlike the other two energy systems, so it uses oxygen.

- The oxidative system is active for most of your day: while sitting at a computer, walking around, and even just watching television. Carbohydrates and fats are the primary fuel sources used to provide ATP in the oxidative system, but this system can also metabolize some protein for energy production. This does not typically happen, though, unless someone has been exercising for a very long time (longer than two to three hours) or for someone who has not eaten in a long time.

- You never *only* use fat or *only* use carbohydrates. The reality is that the fuel used to provide ATP in this energy system is typically a combination of fuels and not an all-or-none kind of action.

Fitness and the Respiratory Exchange Ratio

- The fitter you are, the better you become at using fat as a fuel source. Also, the fitter you are, the better you are at saving your stored glucose or glycogen until you really need it—such as when you pick up the intensity of your exercise. This is just one more reason to consider adding physical activity into your daily lifestyle: It will impact the fuel you use all day long.

- As you exercise and your training status increases, you can increase the number of mitochondria that you have in the cells of the muscles at work. This is called mitochondrial density, and you want it to be high. The mitochondria are the organelles within your cells that help you produce large amounts of ATP, so it makes sense that the more exercise you put into your lifestyle, the better you are at making energy.

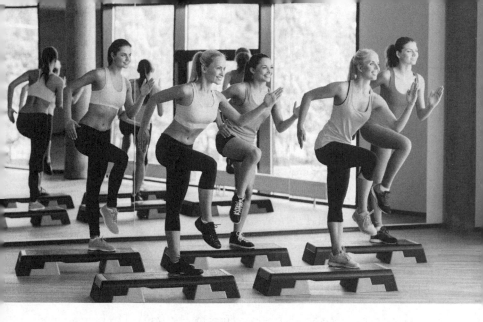

- Another benefit is that you can increase the number of capillaries, or small blood vessels, you have to bring blood, oxygen, and other nutrients to working muscles. This is called capillary density, which you also want to be high.

- Additionally, with exercise training, you actually increase the activity of enzymes called lipases that increase fat breakdown. Exercise also increases the hormones that are used to help initiate this breakdown.

- By making exercise a part of your life, you increase your body's ability to effectively use fuels. You decrease your reliance on carbohydrates and use more fat for fuel, regardless of what you are doing all day. This means that at rest and during exercise, you are burning a greater amount of fat. Over time, this will impact your body composition.

- The fat that is used to make ATP can come from stored fat tissue, such as the fat around your waist and hips, or from dietary fat that you've eaten. You even have fat stored in your muscles to use for energy; this type of fat is called intramuscular triglyceride (IMTG).

- Interestingly, you'll find IMTGs in both very fit people and also out-of-shape people. But how these storage depots of fat are utilized is extremely different between the fit and unfit. For the out-of-shape people, these intramuscular fat stores can do harm and alter the proper cell signaling that should occur in response to various hormones. But in physically active people, the intramuscular fats tend to be used as an energy source, sparing glycogen and increasing fat use for activity.

- So, while both fat and carbohydrates will be used in the oxidative system, the amount of fat used compared to how much carbohydrate used is highly dependent on a number of key factors, including when you last ate, when you last exercised, how fit you are, and what hormones are circulating in your blood.

- The human body is amazing and adjusts to what you eat by burning more of that type of nutrient. This ability to shift easily from one fuel source to another based on the circumstance is called metabolic flexibility.

- In a lab setting, we can determine which fuel source (fat or carbohydrate) you are using by measuring the amounts of carbon dioxide and oxygen in your breath at rest or during exercise. The ratio of carbon dioxide produced to oxygen consumed is called the respiratory exchange ratio (RER). When burning 100 percent fat for fuel, your RER is equal to 0.7, but when burning 100 percent carbohydrate for energy, your RER is 1.

- Basically, the faster and harder you go, the greater percent of carbohydrate that will be used to make energy, or ATP. But there will always be a mix of carbohydrates, fats, and some proteins used to produce ATP. The more metabolically flexible you are, the better you will be at using all the energy sources at the exact right moment.

Try This

Aim to change your food intake and carbohydrate intake based on your activity level each day.

Questions to Consider

1. If you like to walk as your primary form of physical activity, what fuel are you most likely to use to provide energy? What source of food might you want to consider eating more of? Less of?

2. What activities might the first energy system, the creatine phosphate system, be used for in your typical daily routine?

3. How will understanding nutrient bioenergetics impact the choices you will make while trying to improve body composition?

Carbohydrates: Composition, Storage, and Use

I n this lecture, you will learn why carbohydrates—fruit, pasta, whole grains, corn, peas, and breads—don't have to be scary or off-limits. You will also learn how carbohydrates impact your body composition and health, why there might be certain carbohydrates to eat at certain times of the day, and how exercise fits into the puzzle. In the end, you will have a firm grasp of the many types of carbohydrates that exist, how and why they might impact your body composition differently, and when you can eat a high-carbohydrate meal with less fear of storing it as fat.

Glucose and Ketosis

- Glucose is the preferred fuel source by your brain and nervous system, as opposed to protein or fat. The body needs glucose for some actions, and it is estimated that we make about 50 grams of glucose per day in a process called gluconeogenesis. This amount is quite low, and for people who are physically active and like to exercise, the amount of carbohydrate needed will likely be more.

- The current acceptable macronutrient distribution range from the Institute of Medicine for carbohydrate is between 45 and 65 percent of your total calorie intake, with no less than 130 grams of carbohydrate per day to meet our basic physiological needs. Because 1 gram of carbohydrate yields 4 calories, you will need roughly 500 calories per day from carbohydrates just to meet minimal needs.

- However, more and more research is showing that we might be able to consume far less than 130 grams per day as long as dietary fat and protein are increased in the diet.

■ Fortunately, when you eat very little carbohydrate, you can still function from the production of ketones, which are simply a by-product of excess fat breakdown as a result of a low-carbohydrate diet. This excess fat breakdown is called ketosis.

■ Recently, ketone use for energy has been the topic of much research and debate. Some experts support nutritional ketosis for weight loss and health. Nutritional ketosis is induced when a person is put on a low-carbohydrate diet to encourage the breakdown of excess fat. Other experts recommend the traditional model of a higher-carbohydrate, low-fat diet for weight management and health.

■ The research is clear that some glucose is required for life, and even more is likely needed if you decide to become extremely active. However, most scientists agree that the United States is an "over-carbed" nation. They recommend that steps be taken to identify which carbohydrates are best to eat at what times during the day to provide the best health and performance benefits and to minimize negative changes to body composition.

■ How active you are, what size you are, and what your specific goals are will dictate how much carbohydrate you should have in your diet.

■ Of the three macronutrients (carbohydrates, fats, and proteins), carbohydrates are traditionally thought of as the most important fuel for exercise, particularly during high-intensity exercise.

■ The carbohydrate foods that we eat can range from quite simple, like sugar, to more complex forms, like starches and fibers. This ultimately determines how quickly we digest, absorb, and use them to fuel our activity or store them as fat in our muscles, liver, or fat tissue.

Types of Carbohydrates

- We classify carbohydrates by their structure, from simplest to most complex. These include monosaccharides, disaccharides, oligosaccharides, and polysaccharides.

- In all of these types of carbohydrates, the term "saccharide" means "sugar." The prefixes "mono-," "di-," "oligo-," and "poly-" refer to how many sugars are linked together—1, 2, 3 to 9, and 10 or more, respectively.

- The length of the carbohydrate chain is one factor that determines the rate of carbohydrate breakdown. The shorter the chain, the faster this rate becomes. In terms of overall health, you want a slower rate of breakdown to avoid any large variations in blood sugar and insulin concentrations. Insulin is one hormone that is responsible for inhibiting our ability to use fat as a fuel.

- Another interesting factor that determines the rate of carbohydrate breakdown is the shape of the carbohydrate. Starch, which is

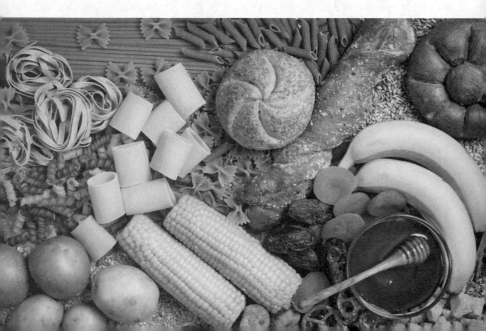

carbohydrate from plant sources, can have two basic forms: amylose (a straight, long chain molecule that is digested slowly) and amylopectin (which is highly branched and rapidly digested). Glycogen is also highly branched and is the form of carbohydrate that we store in our bodies.

- In the context of body composition, we typically just think about the carbohydrates we eat as something that either makes us fat or doesn't. However, we also have to remember that carbohydrates provide us with fuel to ultimately produce energy, especially when we try to exercise at a high intensity.

- Another source of carbohydrate that has clear health and body composition benefits is fiber. Dietary fibers are from plants and are not digested or absorbed by humans, so having these in your diet will slow the rate of carbohydrate digestion, which is usually a good thing.

- Dietary fibers are found in foods like bananas, oatmeal, beans, whole grains, and dark leafy greens.

- Fiber might help you feel more satiated or full for a longer period of time, lower your blood cholesterol and fat levels, and improve overall gut health. That means you might eat less by including fiber in your meals.

Digestion

- The process of carbohydrate breakdown starts in your mouth with an enzyme called salivary amylase. It breaks the long sugars apart into smaller units to be absorbed. These small simple carbohydrates move through the cell lining of the small intestine and into the blood in capillaries that lead to the portal vein.

- The portal vein takes blood to the liver, and the liver takes what glucose it needs for its own energy requirements and also what it needs to store as glycogen.

- The remaining glucose continues to circulate in the blood. No matter what carbohydrate you eat, ultimately it will be in your blood as glucose because your body favors glucose for production of energy, or ATP.

- The fructose you eat is stored as liver glycogen, and once the liver stores all the glycogen it needs from fructose, fructose then serves to increase fat synthesis. Clearly, this might not be the best thing for overall health.

- The end result of carbohydrate breakdown is glucose being directed into circulation and ultimately to the cells that need it throughout your body.

Glycemic Index, Glycemic Load, and Insulin Index

- There is a limit to how much glucose the body can use, and when those uses are met, the body responds by storing the energy in other forms, such as fat.

- The glucose in your blood is used by cells to produce energy, especially by your nervous system and red blood cells.

- Glucose can be stored as glycogen for later use, or the fat cells can remove glucose from the blood to form glycerol that is needed for triglyceride, or fat, storage.

- Our bodies work best for us when blood glucose remains at a constant level without large fluctuations throughout the day. To a large extent, blood glucose levels can determine our mood and energy levels.

- When blood sugar is elevated for a prolonged period of time, numerous detrimental health and body composition outcomes may occur, particularly for people who are hypo- or hyperglycemic. The good thing is that we have an index that tells us how quickly a food you eat will raise your blood glucose levels: the glycemic index.

- By knowing the glycemic index of common foods that you eat, you will have an idea of what your blood glucose response will be after you eat that food. The higher your blood glucose, the higher the hormone insulin is in your blood.

■ Insulin is highly involved with the storage of carbohydrates in your cells. Insulin also blunts fat burning in most cases. It plays a critical role in this important function of balancing blood glucose levels.

■ If you have high insulin levels for a prolonged period of time, losing fat will likely be much more difficult to do. High levels of insulin also might interfere with your ability to achieve optimal health and performance.

■ Foods like bread, pastries, and bagels have a high glycemic index and therefore spike your blood sugar. On the other hand, foods like apples, cherries, beans, and nuts tend to have a much lower glycemic index.

■ The glycemic index provides a snapshot of good information but needs to be balanced with some other basic nutrition principles. One mechanism that has been developed to overcome some of the shortcomings of the glycemic index is called the glycemic load.

■ The glycemic load is the glycemic index of a particular food multiplied by the actual amount of food that you eat. Similar to a high glycemic index, a high glycemic load of a carbohydrate food means that your blood glucose values will increase quickly.

■ This glucose response is used to predict what should happen to insulin levels. The problem is that there is not always a direct correlation between a high glycemic index or a high glycemic load food with a high insulin response.

■ For this reason, research from *The American Journal of Clinical Nutrition* has provided an insulin index of common foods. So, rather than eating and measuring how high glucose gets in your blood, we would measure how high insulin gets in response to specific foods.

■ The glycemic index, glycemic load, and insulin index are useful tools, but other methods for choosing carbohydrates should also be considered. Ideally, we need a way to monitor the carbohydrates that we eat so that they serve the greatest benefit to us while also minimizing any negative impact to our body composition and health.

Balancing Blood Glucose

■ Lower-glycemic-index, lower-glycemic-load, and lower-insulin-index foods have the best potential to improve your body composition, keep you healthy, and avoid large spikes in blood glucose and insulin.

■ On the other hand, many prepackaged foods and other refined carbohydrates will quickly get into your bloodstream and over time have the greatest chance for causing some negative health consequences, including insulin resistance, where your body has to produce more and more insulin just to have the same effect it normally should have.

■ So, unprocessed carbohydrates like vegetables, which are high in fiber and nutrient density, should be the staple of your carbohydrate intake, compared to overly processed carbohydrates and added sugars. Eating this way regularly should improve your fiber and micronutrient intake and increase your feeling of fullness, or satiety, for a longer period of time after eating.

■ Another step in keeping blood glucose levels balanced is to exercise. At the end of exercise, your body is primed to store glucose as glycogen. Additionally, the exercise has increased your body's insulin sensitivity, meaning that you are more responsive to less of this powerful hormone. Theoretically, then, the best time to consume any carbohydrate-heavy meals would be after vigorous exercise, because you are metabolically prepared to handle them best at that point.

Try This

Aim to eat your most starchy meal of the day, such as pasta, after your hardest workouts.

Questions to Consider

1. What sources of carbohydrate in your diet would be best for optimizing your body composition?

2. How many added sugars do you eat on a typical day?

Fat: Not the Nutritional Bad Guy

This lecture focuses on the many different valuable and necessary physiological roles that fat has in the human body. While fat has been maligned as the nutrition "bad guy" for a long time, there is new evidence indicating that eating fat is likely not all that bad for health or body composition, as long as fat intake is not combined with high sugar/refined carbohydrate intake; fat is consumed in a more balanced manner between saturated, monounsaturated, and polyunsaturated fats; and total calorie intake remains aligned with your nutritional and body composition goals.

What Is Fat?

- Just as carbohydrates are composed of monosaccharides linked together, fats are composed of fatty acids. This is the simplest form of fat. And fat goes by a few names. You might hear about fat as a lipid or even a phospholipid. All of these are considered fats, and in general, they are all composed of carbon, hydrogen, and oxygen atoms, just like carbohydrates.

- However, the carbon chain in fats is much longer than the carbon chain in a carbohydrate. This longer carbon chain is a unique feature of fats and plays a pivotal role in energy production. All fats also contain nine calories per gram, making them the macronutrient that provides more calories per gram than any carbohydrate or protein, which both provide only four calories per gram.

- Fatty acids are found in the food you eat. There are two types of fatty acids that you've heard of already: saturated fatty acids and unsaturated fatty acids.

- Fatty acids vary by the length of their carbon-to-carbon chain and the number of hydrogen atoms that surround the carbon chain. That's the definition of saturated or unsaturated fat: They are either saturated with hydrogens or not.

- When fatty acids are joined together, you get a triglyceride. Triglycerides are lipids with three fatty acids that are attached to a glycerol backbone. Triglycerides are the major storage form of fat in the body and the major form of fat in your diet.

- On a food label, you will often see saturated and unsaturated fats highlighted. You might also see monounsaturated, polyunsaturated, and trans fats listed.

- Saturated fats are saturated with hydrogens and have no double bonds in the carbon chain. These fats—like animal fats in meat and butter—are usually solid at room temperature.

- When saturated fats are the predominant source of fat in the diet or just eaten in excess, they have been associated with increased blood levels of total cholesterol. And high cholesterol levels have been correlated in some research to increased risk of heart disease.

- However, new research questions the common recommendation that we need to lower our saturated fat intake from our diets.

- Some experts now suggest that high saturated fat in combination with high intake of sugar and other processed carbohydrates might be the real problem for our health and body composition. In fact, saturated fat might be less of a problem than originally thought, as long as carbohydrate intake is not excessive and a balanced fat intake is in place.

- A balance of fat intake occurs when unsaturated fats are also in your diet. Unsaturated fats contain one or more double bonds along the carbon chain, meaning that, unlike saturated fat, they are not completely saturated with hydrogen molecules.

- There are two types of unsaturated fats: monounsaturated fats and polyunsaturated fats. Monounsaturated fats have only one unsaturated bond (also called a double bond), while polyunsaturated fats have more than one unsaturated (double) bond.

- An easy way to identify an unsaturated fat is that it is typically in liquid form at room temperature. But if unsaturated fats are chilled or refrigerated, they will solidify.

- Examples of monounsaturated fat include olive oil, canola oil, peanut oil, and sesame oil. You will also find monounsaturated fats in foods like avocados, peanut butter, and many nuts and seeds.

- The polyunsaturated fats are also known as essential fatty acids, meaning that they are essential to eat because our bodies cannot make them naturally. Many foods have a mix of fat types, but some examples of polyunsaturated fats include soybean oil, canola oil, flax, tofu, soybeans, and fatty fish like salmon.

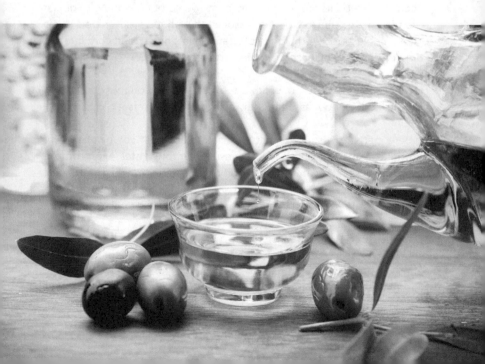

■ Polyunsaturated fats include both omega-6 and omega-3 fatty acids. These essential fatty acids are needed for immune function, vision, and cell membrane integrity, among other things.

Omega-6, Omega-3, and Trans Fat

■ Omega-6 fatty acids ultimately produce compounds that are involved with inflammation, blood vessel constriction, and immunity. All of these functions are important, and it's critical that they are well controlled.

■ Because omega-6 fats lead to inflammation when taken at high levels, they are known as pro-inflammatory agents. Eating too many foods with omega-6 fatty acids, such as heated vegetable oils and many boxed and packaged grocery items, can compromise health and optimal body composition, especially when not balanced with other types of fats, such as omega-3 fatty acids.

■ Omega-3 fatty acids are beneficial for health, due to their anti-inflammatory effects and effects on decreasing blood clot formation. Some omega-3 fatty acids keep cells less rigid and more fluid. In doing so, they promote blood vessel dilation, which lowers blood pressure and can decrease instances of heart attacks.

■ Omega-3 fatty acid consumption can also lower blood concentrations of triglycerides, cut the chances of rheumatoid arthritis, and even reduce some behavioral disorders. Some data even shows that low omega-3 intake is associated with both poor memory and mood disorders.

■ Because omega-3 fatty acids essentially have the opposite role of omega-6 fatty acids, a balanced intake of omega-6 and omega-3 will be needed for optimal health and physical function.

■ Americans tend to have very high omega-6 fatty acid consumption in comparison to omega-3 fatty acids in the diet. This is a problem because a high ratio is reported to promote things like cardiovascular disease, cancer, and inflammatory and autoimmune diseases. But a higher intake of omega-3 fatty acids seems to have the opposite effect and reduce the likelihood of cardiovascular disease, cancer, and inflammatory disorders.

■ If you can't lower your omega-6 intake, then be sure to reduce the gap in the ratio by eating more omega-3 fatty acids. For optimal health, decrease the amount of omega-6 fats that you eat and increase the amount of omega-3 fats that you eat.

■ The other type of fat is trans fat. Trans fats are often in the media, and legislation in the United States to completely ban trans fats from restaurants has been a big issue.

■ Trans fat is made in an industrial manufacturing process that adds hydrogen to previously liquid vegetable oil, making it a solid at room temperature. The fat is essentially artificially hydrogenated.

■ This is done to give foods a longer shelf life and might make certain foods taste better. Many restaurants will use partially hydrogenated vegetable oils to deep-fry foods because the oil does not need to be changed as frequently as other types of oils, resulting in a cost savings.

■ Many foods contain trans fats, including many baked goods, fried foods, potato chips, and margarine. A diet high in trans fats might increase your "bad," or LDL, cholesterol and decrease your "good," or HDL, cholesterol. It might also be associated with your risk of developing heart disease. But some trans fat occurs naturally in food, so it is not entirely avoidable.

How Much Fat Should You Eat?

■ Opinions vary when it comes to how much of each type of fat you should eat. The American Heart Association recommends that, for good health, the majority of the fats that you eat should be monounsaturated or polyunsaturated, rather than saturated fats and trans fats.

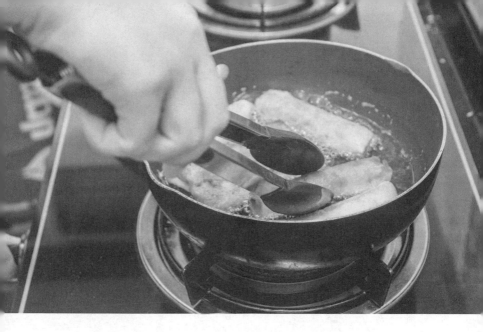

- Others recommend eating about one-third of each type of fat—saturated, monounsaturated, and polyunsaturated fats—that includes a balance of omega-6 and omega-3 fatty acids.

- The 2010 Dietary Guidelines for Americans recommends fat intake between 20 and 35 percent of your total calorie intake and recommends that saturated fat make up no more than 10 percent of these calories. They also recommend replacing "solid fats" with oils when possible and limiting foods with trans fats or hydrogenated oils as much as possible. The guidelines also recommend eating less than 300 milligrams of dietary cholesterol per day.

- Fat is the most energy-dense macronutrient that we eat, because one gram of fat yields nine calories. Many people don't need to seek out additional fat to eat when considering total fat eaten per day, because fat is usually in many of the foods that we eat normally.

- However, research is showing that it might be useful to make an effort to eat more high-quality fats in your diet, such as nuts, seeds, avocados, and fish. These foods provide a nice variety of saturated, monounsaturated, and polyunsaturated fats. And because fats help you feel full, these foods can be used to help reduce the total number of calories that you consume in a day.

Burning Fat

- Fat provides the most abundant source of energy that we have. It fuels your body at rest and during activity that is light to moderate in intensity. During this type of exercise, a muscle's main source of fat supply is your fat (or adipose) tissue.

- Muscles can also rely on fat that is stored inside of the muscle called intramuscular triglycerides (IMTG). The amount of IMTG used during exercise or activity will vary with fitness level. The more fit you are, the more fat you use.

- This is a great adaptation to exercise. With fat stored in your muscle, it is already located where it needs to be so that it can be used as energy. The amount of IMTG will also vary with the intensity and duration of exercise, where longer and slower activity will rely more on fat use than short and fast activity.

- To use fat as a fuel during exercise, your body needs to be able to break down stored triglyceride into free fatty acids to make ATP for energy. The intensity of the exercise will determine if fat will be used during exercise. The more intense the exercise, the less your body will be able to utilize the fat stores, and vice versa.

- Fat oxidation (or burning) is regulated in part by how much glucose you have in your blood. So, eating lots of carbohydrates will increase blood glucose and decrease the breakdown of stored body fat (which is called lipolysis) and fat's use (or oxidation) for energy.

- But fat oxidation is enhanced by exercise training. This occurs because exercise training can increase the number of mitochondria you have, as well as the capillary density. The increase in mitochondria will help the body process the fat at a higher volume, and the increase in capillary density will help increase the blood flow and oxygen delivery to the exercising muscle, which is required to burn fat.

■ Another interesting aspect of fat burning is the differences we see between men and women. Recently, it was reported that fat use relative to total body muscle mass was higher in women than in men. In general, women also tend to have a higher fat oxidation than men during exercise of low to moderate intensity. But women and men alike need to exercise to use fat and to eat in the best possible way to support fat use and optimal health.

Try This

Add at least two servings of fatty fish to your diet each week or begin to use a high-quality fish oil supplement.

Questions to Consider

1. What types of fat do you normally eat? What is in your kitchen now?

2. Does eating fat make you fat?

Protein's Critical Role in Body Composition

E ating more protein might be the best nutritional strategy to manage body composition, given its influence on metabolism, satiety, and even maintenance of muscle mass. And the impact of a high-protein diet when combined with an exercise program can provide even better results for improving our metabolism and body composition. In this lecture, you will learn how protein does all of these positive things in our bodies and how you can use it to improve your body composition.

Protein and Metabolism

- In terms of our body composition, eating protein can help boost your metabolism. In fact, there are a number of foods and supplements that are thought to boost your resting metabolic rate. But exercise and nutrition research suggests that you can do that by including more protein in your diet and by eating lean protein with every meal—such as chicken, turkey breast, fish, and lean beef. Plant protein sources—such as beans, legumes, some grains, and tofu—can be incorporated as well.

- This strategy can be controversial, but much of the current research supports the fact that protein should make up about 20 to 30 percent of your diet. This is higher than the 10 to 15 percent that has been traditionally recommended.

- This recommendation applies to healthy individuals free from kidney disease (because protein could be an added stress to someone with diseased kidneys). Protein is especially important when trying to lose weight.

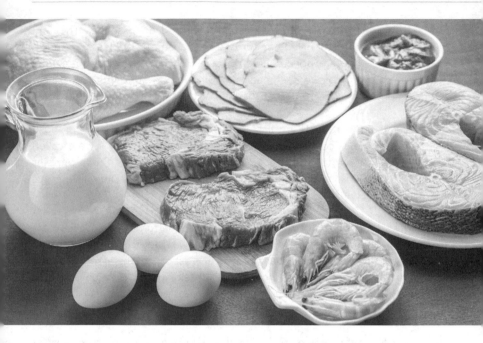

Protein Functions

■ Similar to carbohydrates and fats, proteins contain carbon, hydrogen, and oxygen, but proteins also have a nitrogen molecule attached to their structure. It is this nitrogen found in protein that distinguishes it from the other macronutrients.

■ Proteins are composed of amino acids that are linked together by peptide bonds. Twenty different amino acids exist, and they can all combine in unique ways to make new and different proteins in our bodies.

■ But because so many different types of foods can provide you with protein, how can you tell if a specific protein or protein food is good-quality protein? One way to tell is by knowing the biological value of the protein. The higher the biological value of a protein, the higher its quality.

- There are two types of proteins: essential and nonessential. They are either essential to include in our diets because our bodies don't make them, or they are nonessential because our bodies make them from other proteins, so we don't need to worry about eating them. There are 11 nonessential and 9 essential amino acids.

- Essential amino acids are the ones we tend to worry about the most. When proteins contain all of the essential amino acids, they are called "complete" proteins and have a high biological value. These proteins are typically from animal sources and include meat, poultry, fish, eggs, milk, and cheese.

- When food does not have all of the essential amino acids, they are called "incomplete" proteins and have a low biological value. These are lower-quality proteins that are missing at least one of the essential amino acids. A diet made up of incomplete proteins might eventually lead to protein malnutrition. Examples of incomplete proteins are usually found in plants, grains, nuts, and vegetables.

- Classifying the amino acids like this is probably most important for people who do not eat animal products. This is because animal meats contain all of the essential amino acids, but plant products generally do not. This means that one or more of the amino acids will be missing, which could mean that you won't be able to make certain products that your body needs.

- The good news is that most people don't eat only one source of plant food. And by combining various types of incomplete proteins, you can make up for any amino acids that were missing in your diet. This is called eating complementary proteins. The most common example of this is to eat rice and beans together.

- One exception is soy, which is a plant product that *does* contain all of the essential amino acids, making it a complete protein.

- Of the 9 essential amino acids, three are important because they are branched-chain amino acids, which can provide some fuel during long bouts of exercise or when we go long periods of time between eating. They might also help improve body composition.

- The three branched-chain amino acids are leucine, isoleucine, and valine. These amino acids have a "branched" side chain that distinguishes them from other amino acids.

- If you work out, consuming branched-chain amino acids might be beneficial in preventing muscle damage or helping repair damaged muscle tissue. This means that you might be less sore and uncomfortable after moderate to strenuous exercise if protein—such as milk, yogurt, or a protein shake—is consumed beforehand.

- With regard to body composition, leucine gets the most attention of the three because it is considered to be the "trigger" to start muscle protein synthesis. In fact, research suggests that you not only want to eat some protein at each meal, but that you might also want to make sure that you are getting roughly two to three grams of leucine in the protein foods that you eat.

- Over the past 5 to 10 years, there has been a huge increase in scientific papers that support using protein or amino acids to prevent the loss of muscle as a result of aging or extreme exercise. The scientific literature has repeatedly shown that a higher-protein diet helps with fat loss and improves body composition.

Nitrogen Balance

- Some amino acids, such as the branched-chain amino acids and alanine, can be used to make ATP in your energy systems. In this way, it is estimated that protein contributes as much as 10 to 15 percent of your energy supply during intense prolonged exercise.

- One common way to use amino acids for energy is to convert them to glucose in a process called the glucose-alanine cycle. This is one way to produce new glucose from non-carbohydrate sources, which is known as gluconeogenesis. This is how the amino acid alanine contributes to energy production.

- Research shows that the more oxygen a person consumes, such as when breathing heavily from exercise, the greater the amount of leucine she or he uses as a fuel source.

- In the process of eating protein, using it to make other proteins, and using it for energy, proteins are constantly being broken down (or metabolized) and built back up (or synthesized). This process is called protein turnover, and it is a never-ending process, which is why we must eat a sufficient amount of protein in our diets, particularly when we exercise a lot.

- Nitrogen is the part of protein that distinguishes it from carbohydrates and fat on a chemical level. In the lab, we can measure nitrogen balance, which is the balance between nitrogen intake and nitrogen output. Protein foods can be analyzed for their nitrogen content, and this will take care of the "nitrogen in" part of the nitrogen balance equation. Doctors can then analyze nitrogen from body outputs, including urine, feces, sweat, skin, and hair.

- When nitrogen intake is higher than output, you are in a positive nitrogen balance. In this scenario, you would likely be "anabolic" and in a muscle growth mode. If you are trying to maintain or build muscle mass, or lose fat, you want to be in a positive nitrogen balance.

- When nitrogen intake is less than nitrogen output, you are in negative nitrogen balance. In this case, you would likely be sacrificing muscle to support your protein needs. This occurs during very long and intense workouts, if you don't eat for very long periods of time, or during the normal process of aging—if you don't pay attention to how much protein you eat.

■ States of positive and negative nitrogen balance are drastically different and are both very important to your overall body composition.

■ Factors that might affect nitrogen balance include protein quality and total calorie intake. High-quality animal proteins, such as eggs and dairy products, are best because of their amino acid content and high digestibility—that is, they are easy to digest and absorb.

■ Plant proteins have lower digestibility—meaning that they are more difficult to digest and absorb and are low in some essential amino acids. In fact, a common recommendation for vegetarians is to increase protein intake by about 10 percent, just to account for this.

Exercise and Protein Needs

■ The amount of protein in your diet can make a difference to overall body composition and health, but protein needs can change based on how much and what type of exercise you do.

■ Endurance and resistance exercise can use or burn a lot of calories. This fact alone would require more protein in your diet, but exercise also puts a lot of strain on your body's protein stores.

■ Protein breakdown increases when you exercise hard, and protein intake at an optimal level is required to maintain or improve muscle mass. Ultimately, you have the best chance at maintaining or improving muscle mass by choosing a diet with high rather than adequate protein levels.

Metabolism and Energy Balance

■ There are three major components of total daily energy expenditure: resting metabolic rate, the thermic effect of activity, and the thermic effect of food. The largest percent of total daily energy expenditure belongs to our resting metabolic rate—close to 75 percent.

- Your metabolism tends to slow as you age. The overall decrease in metabolism is only about one to three percent during the aging process, which really isn't much and can be offset with a few simple nutrition or exercise strategies—one of which might be eating more protein.

- How does eating more protein help us adjust to a slowing metabolism? Your body digests a certain percentage of the macronutrients we eat—protein, carbohydrates, and fat—and protein is the least digested, because your body cannot oxidize, or burn, the nitrogen in protein sources of food.

- In essence, your body works hard to digest and absorb protein, and this is probably why eating protein gives you the largest increase in metabolism when eating it. This is called the thermic effect of food. A

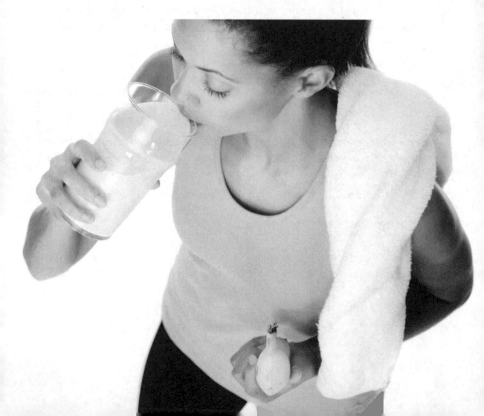

number of research studies have been designed to measure metabolism after a meal containing protein versus fat versus carbohydrate, and the majority of these indicate that the greatest increase in metabolism comes after eating protein.

- In addition to the increase in metabolism we get from eating protein, it also makes us feel the most satiated after eating it. Here, the research is also clear: Low protein intake is linked to increased feelings of hunger and desire to eat again, while increased protein intake is linked to decreased feelings of hunger and less desire to eat again.

- Even without exercise, research is showing that adding protein to the diet of overweight (but otherwise healthy) people can help improve body composition.

How Much Protein Do You Need?

- The standard recommendation for protein is 0.8 grams per kilogram (0.36 grams per pound) of body weight per day, but we need more to have an optimal body composition response. The most recent research tells us we should be consuming up to about double the current recommendation.

- Most women can aim for about one palm-sized portion of protein every time you eat. Most men can aim for two palm-sized portions of protein at each meal. This will, surprisingly, come close to your optimal needs for protein without having to count and weigh everything you eat.

- These guidelines should be discussed with a qualified professional to get specific recommendations. You want information that best suits your lifestyle and health status.

Try This

Make sure you make protein a priority with every meal.

Questions to Consider

1. How much protein do you need to add to your diet to meet the "new" research recommendations?

2. What food sources of protein are in your diet, and which ones do you want to add to your diet? Why?

High-Protein Diets and Anabolic Resistance

How much protein should you eat? In this lecture, you will learn about the amounts, timing, and type of protein that you might need to consume to lose body fat while maintaining muscle mass—even with a low-calorie diet. You will also learn about muscle growth and breakdown and how, as you grow older, you will need even more protein to support what is happening to your body. In general, diets that are higher than typically recommended in protein are safe and are an effective tool for improving body composition.

The Amount of Protein You Eat

- Many people still think that eating protein will somehow automatically add muscle and make them bigger. This is just not accurate—or gaining muscle would be much easier.

- When people start a diet or purposefully eat less food, one of the major risks is losing muscle mass. You'll lose body weight, but you might also lose a lot of muscle. And that, of course, is a problem because having muscle helps you burn calories, stay active, and be healthy.

- The research to date says that you can preserve muscle mass and decrease fat mass even with severe caloric restriction.

- The ability to maintain muscle while losing fat is one way to rescue our resting metabolism so that it doesn't drop too drastically. This means that you just increased your ability to fight weight regain, or putting all of the weight back on, as is typical after the diet stops or changes.

- When lowering your calorie intake in an attempt to lose body fat, you increase your chances of success by increasing, not decreasing, protein in your diet.

- During calorie restriction, a shift to increase the number of calories you get from protein—which would replace many of the calories you get from carbohydrates and fats—will improve body composition. Even supplementing with milk has been shown to improve body composition when trying to lose weight.

- In terms of recommended amounts, it looks like about two times the recommended dietary allowances can cover most of your bases. That would be about 1.6 grams per kilogram of body weight, or 0.72 grams of protein per pound.

Aging and Anabolic Resistance

- Research shows that people who add more protein to their diets tend to improve their body composition, particularly when exercise is also included. But what about the massive amounts of muscle that we risk losing as we age?

- If you don't work to keep your muscle mass, you will lose muscle mass every decade after about 30 years old. The health implications and your ability to just move around depend on keeping some of your muscle mass.

- When we talk about muscle protein balance, it is important to talk about both the synthesis part, which is known as anabolism (or muscle growth), and the degradation part, known as catabolism (or muscle breakdown). If synthesis matches degradation, you would not gain or lose any muscle. If, however, degradation is greater than synthesis, you would be losing muscle.

- Additionally, certain changes occur that make it more difficult for an older adult to use protein to build or maintain muscle mass. The body

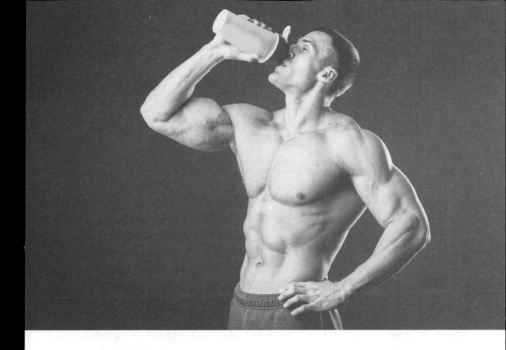

actually starts to resist anabolism, or growth, with age. This process has been coined "anabolic resistance."

- Interestingly, even after consuming an amount of protein that is known to increase muscle protein synthesis, the synthesis response is lower in older adults compared to younger adults. So, even though you hear about a specific protein intake—such as 0.8 grams per kilogram of body mass per day—that is recommended to avoid disease states or muscle wasting, it is much too low to actually optimally improve body composition, especially as you age.

- If you are 20 years old and you eat or drink about 20 to 25 grams of protein following a workout, you will likely maximize your immediate ability to make new muscle proteins. But you need almost twice this amount (that is, about 40 grams) after exercise when you are older to have the same result as seen in younger people. It is probably quite variable at what age this occurs, but you might consider increasing your after-exercise protein intake after about age 40.

- A recent scientific review paper pointed out a number of reasons for why this anabolic resistance might occur as we age, including decreased digestion and absorption of protein, decreased ability for your muscles to absorb amino acids, and decreased anabolic signaling once the protein is eaten.

- This anabolic resistance in older, healthy adults can be overcome with a higher intake of dietary protein. The entire process for muscle repair, maintenance, and growth is blunted as we age. You might just need an extra push—such as more protein—to have the response you want.

- How much protein should you be consuming to keep your muscle protein synthesis high? One study gave healthy older men 10, 20, or 35 grams of whey protein and found that absorption and muscle protein synthesis was greater with 35 grams compared to 10 and 20 grams.

- It looks like there is some sort of anabolic threshold when we talk about protein intake that simply rises as we get older, and that threshold needs to be met to stimulate a response.

- An increased protein intake seems to have a long-term effect, as well. Research has shown that more protein in older people help them maintain their muscle mass better than lower protein intake. Overall, if you are an older adult, every time you eat, think about including a lean protein source of food.

Recommendations for Protein Consumption

- Unfortunately, the recommendations for daily protein consumption vary across organizations. The American College of Sports Medicine recommends 10 to 35 percent of your total calorie intake to come from protein—which equates to about 200 to 700 calories in a standard 2,000-calorie diet. They also recommend increasing protein intake to 1 gram per kilogram of body weight around age 50 and increasing even further in active older individuals.

■ But if you are very active, then how much do you need? The International Society of Sports Nutrition recommends 1.4 to 2 grams of protein per kilogram of body weight for active individuals to improve training adaptations to exercise. This is strongly endorsed by the most current research.

■ Other leading international organizations, such as the Academy of Nutrition and Dietetics and the European Society for Clinical Nutrition and Metabolism, recommend somewhere between 1 and 1.7 grams of protein per kilogram of body weight, depending on your activity level and health status. Overall, recommendations are beginning to increase.

Frequency of Eating and Nighttime Eating

■ The concept of when we eat and at what frequency we should eat is called nutrient timing.

■ When do you want to eat? If you like breakfast or a late-night snack, then eating at those times will probably help you stick to the plan. However, the food you pick to eat at those times will make the difference in how your body ultimately stores the energy.

MYTH
Too Much Protein Is Harmful

A myth about eating too much protein is that it will cause your kidneys to shut down, but this is incorrect. There is a lot of research support for a higher-protein diet; studies show no evidence of kidney disease resulting from eating more protein.

On a high-protein diet, your kidneys do perform more work to handle the protein. However, increased action does not equal damage. This is because—like all of our other bodily functions—the kidneys are very good at adapting.

Overall, there is no overwhelming evidence that says that protein harms the body, but anything in excess can potentially be damaging.

- How should your daily protein needs be split up over a day for the best results? Eating about 20 grams of protein per meal, spaced evenly throughout the day, is commonly recommended. The research here is mixed, though.

- Unfortunately, research shows that older individuals typically consume 8 grams of protein at breakfast, 12 grams of protein at lunch, and a maximum of 40 grams of protein at dinner. This type of spread of protein is considered protein back-loading. It is very common, but for optimal results, it seems that the dose of protein should be spaced a bit more evenly throughout the day, to stimulate muscle protein synthesis.

- In overweight and obese older individuals, evenly spaced protein stimulates muscle protein synthesis significantly more effectively than this back-loaded practice. Interestingly, when resistance training is added, muscle protein synthesis normalizes no matter how the protein is eaten. Back-loaded or not, resistance training improves how we respond to eating.

- If you simply don't like eating frequently, you can also have great results by eating less frequently. You just need to be sure that when you do eat, you're eating nutrient-dense foods and getting high-quality protein in those foods.

- Another time of day that people often want to eat is before bed. It might actually be good for you to eat a small protein snack or drink a protein shake before bed.

- When young and older men were given 40 grams of casein protein before bed, their muscle protein synthesis was significantly higher overnight than when they drank a no-calorie drink, regardless of their age.

- How do other macronutrients and other forms of protein—besides casein—eaten or consumed before bed affect metabolism and health? In one study, the effect of a nighttime snack on next-day resting metabolic rate was influenced by the sex, age, and fitness level of the person.

- What about the effect of nighttime eating on body composition? The first study to look at 12 weeks of nighttime eating before sleep and exercise training found that by simply drinking a protein shake before sleep, muscle size was improved, and so was strength.

- It looks like very small, 150-calorie protein drinks before bed might actually be advisable, rather than something to avoid, but much more research is needed in this area.

Protein Powders

- It can be difficult to eat a lot of high-protein meals. It just makes you feel very full. So, an easy way to add extra protein is in the form of protein powders. There are many types of protein powders on the market.

- There are many forms of protein. Whey protein isolate is considered the purest form of protein. Hydrolyzed whey protein isolate is the most expensive because of the purity and the processes involved to make it. Whey protein concentrate has less filtering and therefore more natural carbohydrates and fats from milk, making the protein content lower in most cases—about 35 to 80 percent protein.

- Two other very common sources and types of protein powders are casein, also from milk, and soy protein. Although these proteins also increase muscle protein synthesis, whey is usually considered best for improving muscle protein synthesis, especially post-workout. This is because of whey's higher leucine content—the essential branched-chain amino acid that contributes the most to muscle protein synthesis.

- Casein and soy are good options, though, for people who just don't like whey, for those who want something that is slower digesting (casein), or for vegetarians (soy).

- Many other sources also exist, such as hemp, pea, and even bug proteins, but less research exists on those.

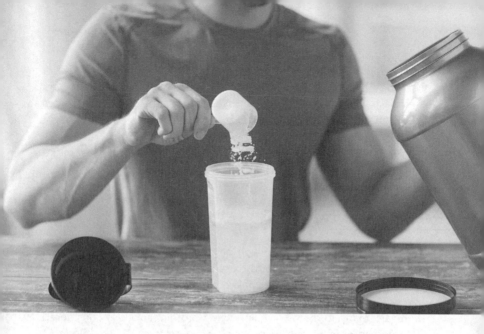

- Milk is also an acceptable source of protein and has been found to increase lean body mass more than soy protein after 12 weeks of a resistance-training program. But milk also has both carbohydrates and fat in it.

- What do you look for on the label of a supplement? You want the highest percent of protein per scoop. You ideally want a powder with more than 80 percent protein in each scoop.

- Take caution, though, when reading the labels on protein powders. Many powders have added proteins that our body cannot use toward building muscle—even if they contribute to the total nitrogen content. Some examples of protein fillers are l-glycine and l-taurine. Supplement companies cleverly market these fillers to make them look like they will help you, but they probably won't.

- Overall, protein powders can be a great, convenient way to increase protein intake, and most of them taste great. You can't beat the great effects on body composition with the addition of this supplement to your diet.

Try This

Experiment with protein powders to find one that makes it convenient for you to take in enough protein to optimize your body composition.

Questions to Consider

1. What myths were busted in this lecture?

2. What foods do you eat that contribute to your daily protein needs?

Critical Micronutrients and Water

I n this lecture, you will learn about what vitamins and minerals are, some specific roles that vitamins and minerals have in your body, what foods make up good sources of some of the major micronutrients, and how to recognize both deficiencies and overloading toxicities that can occur with specific micronutrients. To achieve balance, you should aim to add more nutrient-dense foods like vegetables, fruits, and whole grains to your diet; stay active; and take a multivitamin.

Vitamins

■ Micronutrients include both vitamins and minerals. They do not directly provide energy but play a big role in energy production. Micronutrients are needed only in small quantities, so even small fluctuations of higher or lower intake can have a large impact on body composition, health, and performance.

■ Vitamins serve many important functions in our bodies and are involved in digestion, absorption, energy production, antioxidant purposes, and growth. They are regulators in numerous metabolic reactions that release energy from food or help with energy transfer to produce ATP, the energy currency of our bodies.

■ Vitamins are termed "organic compounds" because they contain carbon, just like all three of the macronutrients: carbohydrates, fats, and proteins. Vitamins also act as cofactors and coenzymes, which are required for various interactions in our metabolic pathways.

- For a compound to be considered a vitamin, almost all textbooks will define them as follows.
  - ◆ Vitamins are natural components of foods, usually present in very small amounts.
  - ◆ Vitamins are essential for normal physiological function.
  - ◆ Vitamins, when absent from the diet, will cause a specific deficiency in that particular vitamin.

- This means that you must get vitamins from the food you eat.

- Vitamins are classified as either fat-soluble or water-soluble, depending on whether they dissolve in fat or water. Fat-soluble vitamins include vitamins A, D, E, and K. The body absorbs them from the gastrointestinal tract and stores them in the liver, fatty tissues, and parts of your cells that contain fat, such as the cell membrane.

- Fat-soluble vitamins move in your blood bound to dietary fat. This means that if fat is not part of your diet, you will likely have suboptimal fat absorption and might be set up for a fat-soluble vitamin deficiency. Fat-soluble vitamins are not readily excreted and are stored in your fat cells and liver.

- Water-soluble vitamins include the B vitamins and vitamin C. These vitamins are also absorbed from the gastrointestinal tract and must be transported in the blood with what are called carrier proteins.

- Water-soluble vitamins are not stored in large amounts in the body because body water turnover is so constant. They are also easily excreted through urine and a little bit through your sweat. Because they are so easily excreted and not stored, a daily intake of less than 50 percent of any of the water-soluble vitamins can lead to deficiency in about four weeks.

- This means that if you are missing an entire food group, such as carbohydrates or fats (which can easily happen if you follow a fad diet), it would be fairly easy to be deficient in some vitamins.

- Both deficiencies and toxicities are possible with vitamins. A deficiency is not enough; a toxicity is too much.

- Toxicity is not likely to occur from food alone; it's more common when people are taking supplements. So, don't take more than the recommended dose of whatever supplements you choose to take, and talk to a professional about what you are taking and how much.

- Both deficiencies and toxicities are more likely with certain vitamins and minerals than others. Fat-soluble vitamins are stored more efficiently in the body (there is less fat turnover compared to water turnover). Vitamin A toxicity is the most common form of fat-soluble vitamin toxicity, because it can occur when intake exceeds just two times the needed recommendations.

- When vitamin A accumulates in the liver, you can have both acute and more chronic outcomes. Headache, rashes, visual changes, bone pain, skin cracking, mouth ulcers, yellowing of the skin, nausea, and vomiting are acute outcomes that may occur. Chronic toxicity can even lead to liver damage.

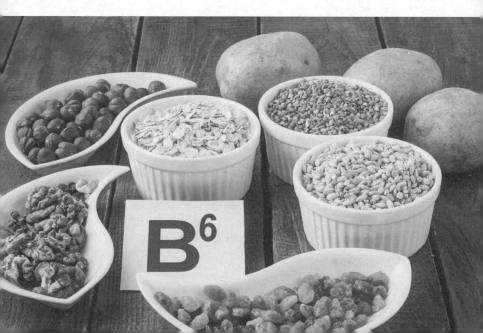

■ Although there is a word of caution about foods containing vitamin A, you should not be afraid to consume them. Just be aware of how much vitamin A you are consuming.

■ Water-soluble vitamins, on the other hand, are much less likely to lead to toxicity, but it could occur from overconsumption of niacin, B_6, and vitamin C. Toxicities are far less common from whole-food choices than from supplements, such as multivitamins.

■ A number of things can impact our overall vitamin needs, such as exercise, stress, aging, sex, and medications. Micronutrient needs will vary from person to person, and a one-size-fits-all approach is not possible.

■ Another interesting note about vitamins is that their status in foods can change just by how you store food and cook food. Poor storage and preparation of food can result in a decreased vitamin content in your food.

■ Things like excessive cooking and exposure to light, heat, air, and water can all lower the vitamin content of foods. Generally, it is best to consume food soon after harvest or buy foods that have been frozen quickly after harvest. The sooner that a fresh fruit or vegetable is frozen, the more vitamin content that will be preserved.

Minerals

■ Minerals are inorganic molecules (meaning molecules without carbon). Like vitamins, they are essential—in very small amounts—and they must be included in our diets because we don't make them naturally.

■ Similar to vitamins, minerals also serve many different regulatory functions in our bodies. They work as cofactors, meaning that they assist enzymes in energy transformation, contribute to production of other cells and enzymes, and help form red blood cells and bones. Minerals are involved in nerve impulses, body growth and development, water balance, muscle movement, and metabolism.

- Electrolytes are minerals that keep our nervous system firing properly. They are electrically charged particles that most commonly include calcium, sodium, potassium, magnesium, and chloride. They help with establishing the electrochemical gradient across cells, which is necessary for proper nerve communication.

- Electrolytes also assist with muscle contraction and modulate fluid exchange within the body's fluid compartments. That means that the electrolyte minerals play a big role in how we store water and where we store water. In this way, they influence our body composition and our body's water content quite a bit.

- Because we need minerals in very small amounts, it is even more critical not to underestimate the value they have for our bodies.

- The two types of minerals are major minerals (also called macrominerals) and trace minerals (also called microminerals). The major minerals include calcium, phosphorus, sodium, and magnesium, and they are required in amounts greater than 100 milligrams per day.

- Trace minerals, on the other hand, include minerals like selenium, iron, and zinc. These are required in amounts less than 100 milligrams per day, and typically even less than 15 milligrams per day.

- Ingestion of a mineral-containing food does not necessarily translate to 100 percent absorption of the mineral. This concept is called mineral bioavailability. In other words, even though you consume food with minerals, there are several factors that can affect how much of this mineral is actually absorbed from the gut to the blood stream.

- In general, there are four factors involved in mineral bioavailability.
  1. *The type of food that contains the minerals.* Typically, animal sources have a better bioavailability of minerals than plant sources.
  2. *Mineral-to-mineral interactions.* Because minerals tend to move through similar receptors in the gastrointestinal tract, high amounts of one mineral may inhibit, or slow down, absorption of another mineral.

3. *Vitamin-mineral interactions.* A positive interaction example is that vitamin C intake improves iron absorption. A dietician will have additional information about foods you can pair to optimize your supplementation strategies for minerals.

4. *Fiber-mineral interaction.* Fiber can bind to minerals and block or slow their absorption. Typically, our dietary fiber comes from plant sources (this is another reason that animal sources might often be superior in terms of mineral bioavailability).

- Consider the food's nutrient density, or how many nutrients it has, compared to its calorie content when you purchase food to eat.

Phytochemicals

- Another component of nutrition that is often considered along with micronutrients is phytochemicals, which are biologically active compounds found in plants that provide zero calories or direct energy but can influence your overall health. Currently, only a few of an extensive list of known phytochemicals have been studied.

- Phytochemicals have numerous roles but are most often linked to disease prevention. They can function as antioxidants that reduce damage caused by reactive oxygen species, can have hormonelike actions, and can even be considered metabolic boosters.

Food Sources versus Dietary Supplements

- Most experts will recommend getting most of your micronutrients from food sources instead of dietary supplements. Research shows that vitamins and minerals from whole foods might have more health benefits than getting the same micronutrients from a supplement.

- Although the reason why is not entirely understood, it is thought that the different types of nutrients in whole foods might interact in a synergistic manner that results in the greater absorption of combined micronutrients than when those micronutrients are taken as a separate

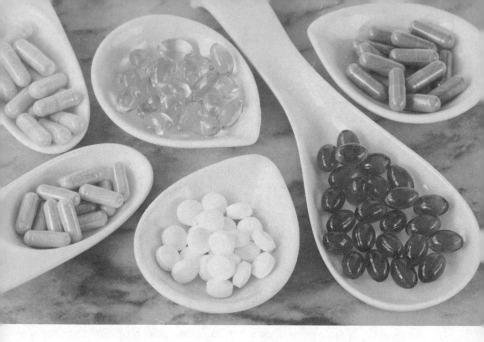

supplement or with a combined multivitamin. Also, there seem to be nutrients that just can't be reproduced in dietary supplements.

■ Some research also shows that single-nutrient supplements can have adverse effects—such as a higher risk of toxicity or possibly just a nutrient-nutrient interaction that might unfavorably impact nutrient absorption—even though intentions were good.

■ So, a diet that includes all the macronutrients from whole foods is most likely the best option, and the best place to start, to get the best micronutrient content out of your food. In addition, you'll likely get other active compounds, such as phytonutrients, by eating a diet consisting mostly of whole foods.

■ The problem is that many people don't eat enough variety of nutrient-dense whole foods in their day-to-day eating. Instead, whole foods get replaced by heavily processed foods for a majority of meals and snacks.

- Over time, nutrient deficiencies can come about by relying solely or mostly on these processed and easily accessed foods. Although many processed foods are appealing and convenient, it is probably a good idea to limit them as much as we can.

- A low-quality diet can lead to nutrient deficiencies, and deficiencies can lead not only to more than just poor health, but they have also been linked to a greater risk of becoming obese. In addition, if you throw deficiency issues on top of hard exercise training, which can also lead to a greater need for certain nutrients, you could be at a huge risk for deficiency.

The Importance of Water

Water is essential for optimal health and body composition, but many people walk around with less-than-adequate hydration levels. In addition to keeping you hydrated, water helps transport all of the nutrients in your body and helps move metabolic waste products out of your body. Water also plays a huge part in the regulation of body temperature, particularly with exercise.

Aim for about 8 to 10 cups, or about 2 liters, of water per day in addition to eating plenty of fruits and vegetables, which are loaded with water.

- Given the prevalence of these vitamin and mineral deficiencies, should you take a vitamin and mineral supplement? It depends. Quite a few people would benefit from taking a multivitamin/multimineral supplement. However, supplementation will not fix a broken diet. Work for a highly nutritious diet first, and then simply use supplements to supplement that diet.

- Also, the recommended intakes for vitamins and minerals were established to only prevent against any deficiencies. They don't consider the achievement of optimal health or body composition.

- To determine if supplementation might help you, think about how many times you eat per day, what quality of food you generally eat, what medications you take, and how much exercise you do on a daily basis. Then, discuss these factors and concerns with your doctor to decide what is right for you.

Try This

Practice drinking 8 to 10 cups of water per day and monitor your urine color.

Questions to Consider

1. What are the main reasons for vitamins and minerals in the body?

2. What does the research say about micronutrient deficiencies in the United States?

Food Labeling and Nutritional Choices

What are the rules that we should follow in the grocery store? How can we decipher a food label and know what we're looking for? What can we identify as important for improving body composition, recovery, or optimal aging? There is no perfect formula, magic food group, or even cursed aisle in the supermarket. Rather, there are bad options, better options, and the best options. In this lecture, you will learn how much food to consume each day, what your dietary intake should look like, and how to interpret each section of the Nutrition Facts label.

How Much Food Should You Eat?

- How much food should you eat? It depends on who you are, how old you are, how big or small you are, how much muscle you have, what your sex is, and what goals you have. These basic indicators will dictate the energy requirements of your body in general.

- At different stages in our lives, we have different energy demands—that is, different amounts of calories that we need to live optimally. For example, a child is constantly growing and developing until the onset of puberty. In comparison to their size, a child will likely require more calories than an adult while they are growing so fast.

- A larger person—in terms of body size, not fat mass—is going to require more absolute energy each day than a smaller person, assuming equal activity levels.

- Men tend to be larger than women. Therefore, based on the previous principle of body size alone, men will often require greater calorie intake than women. However, a second factor is that, on average, men will have

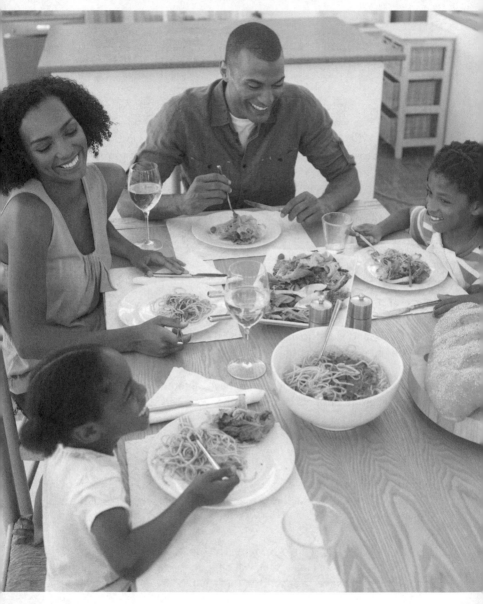

more muscle mass than women. Muscle tissue is highly metabolically active and demands a high energy intake—to keep us moving.

■ Your relative activity level also determines how much food you need to eat every day. If you exercise a lot, you will probably need more food to refuel and recover. But there are also times when you would not want to replenish your energy stores completely.

■ The food you require depends on your goals. Are you trying to lose weight? Or are you trying to put on 5 pounds (2.27 kilograms) of muscle mass? In both of these cases, total caloric intake will be different, and so will the components of that caloric intake.

■ Another area we cannot ignore is genetics. For example, do you have a tendency to gain weight or lose weight easily, and what does your family look like? Answers to these questions are important. However, even a lousy or a fantastic genetic predisposition must be massaged by the other factors that we can control.

■ On nutrition labels, certain nutrients are "based on a 2,000-calorie diet." Not everyone eats a 2,000-calorie diet; this just reflects the caloric intake of an average-sized person to maintain weight and serves as a basic starting point for most people. The percentages listed on the Nutrition Facts label must be adjusted case by case.

Are All Calories Created Equal?

■ Is a calorie just a calorie, regardless of if it's 200 calories of pizza or 200 calories of broccoli? If you consumed primarily calories from simple sugars each day, you might not gain any weight overall, but you would be missing a ton of the nutrients that your body requires to function well, and over time, this would alter your body composition and health for the worse.

■ Importantly, the readout on your scale probably won't change— and you might go on thinking that all is well—but internally the story could be much different. Chances are good that you would develop compromised metabolic, immune, and inflammatory function that, at best, would not allow you to function optimally and, at worst, could lead to serious conditions, such as blood glucose and lipid abnormalities and possibly chronic disease.

■ While we need to be aware of the number of calories we eat, it is probably more important to worry about the quality of those calories. Essentially, eating nutrient-dense foods provides much more bang for your buck. In fact, you often have to eat quite a bit of the quality foods to meet your calorie needs—so you really can eat more and weigh less.

Nutritional Information Labels

■ The first thing to look for on a nutritional label is the serving size, located in the top-left corner of the label. The serving size is important because this is the portion that all the nutritional information is based on. If you choose to eat more or less than the serving size listed, your nutritional intake will also be higher or lower for all nutrients.

■ Next, examine the total number of calories for the given serving size, located at the top of the label. This gives you an idea of how much this product is going to contribute to your entire day's intake. Even though the quantity of calories is less important than the quality of calories, at some point you need to be aware of calories and make sure that you're not eating too many or too few to support your goals.

■ Just below where the total calories are listed is the list of nutrients provided per serving, including total fat and types of fat, cholesterol, sodium, carbohydrates and sugars, and protein. All the values are given in grams and also as a percent daily value, which provides consumers with a general estimate of how much this serving of this particular food will contribute to overall recommendations for each nutrient each day based on a 2,000-calorie diet.

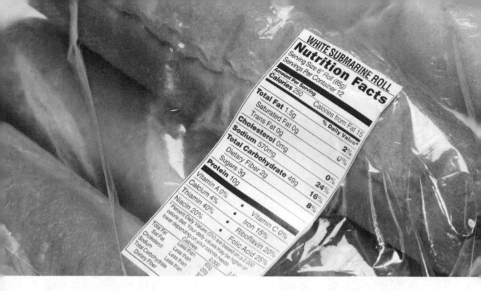

- At the bottom of the food label are the amounts of certain vitamins and minerals, such as vitamin A and C, calcium, and iron. This gives you a better idea of the nutrient density of the food you choose to eat. You should choose higher values of these nutrients paired with a lower-calorie amount on the label.

- The food label is typically paired with a list of ingredients contained in the product. The higher up on the list, the greater relative amount of the ingredient in the food. The first item listed has the greatest relative amount in the food. You want to see more "natural" or unprocessed ingredients toward the beginning of the list.

- It's a good idea to choose foods with as few ingredients as possible to have a better idea of how processed the food is. Today, almost everything is processed to some degree—this is usually for food safety—so choose foods that are as minimally processed as you can.

- The food label—specifically, the ingredients list—is also great if you need to identify anything that could trigger a known allergy. If you are unsure about a food or a name on the label, it's better to stick with the motto of "when in doubt, leave it out."

- The U.S. Food and Drug Administration proposed a change to the label. The new label was proposed to identify a few things.
  - Serving sizes are listed bigger and bolder; they are also updated to reflect more realistic serving sizes.
  - The calories will be listed in a larger font.
  - Added sugars must be listed on the label.
  - There will be other small changes to reflect current nutrition and food science.

Food Labels: Making Good Decisions

- Knowing the food label language will only help you make more consistently good decisions for what to buy and eat if you take a little time to look at the label and interpret whether the food has the nutritional makeup and quality to meet your goals.

- You should also have an idea of what the recommended ranges are for you to try and eat of each nutrient based on things like your age, weight, and sex. But keep in mind that current science continues to update the recommendations that you should follow.

- Let's go through a food label and consider some very general rules of thumb.
  - Make sure to get the right amount of protein in your diet. Determine your protein needs based on factors like age, sex, and your goals. Most people will fall somewhere between 1 and 1.5 grams of protein per kilogram of body mass for protein needs. Then, read the Nutrition Facts label to see how much protein you are eating with each meal. Add up the grams of protein and multiply by 4— the conversion factor for protein grams to protein calories.
  - Use the Nutrition Facts label to look at your carbohydrate intake. Try to limit the amount of simple sugars you eat or drink, and choose more complex starches instead—foods like vegetables and whole grains, which usually have more fiber, too.

◆ On the food label, compare the total carbohydrate value to the amount of sugar and fiber in the product. Is there a high amount of sugar compared to the total carbohydrate value? If so, this is probably a simple carbohydrate that should be limited. A food that has a high amount of fiber and low amount of sugar compared to the total carbohydrate in the product is probably the better day-to-day option.

◆ Some recent research shows that we might be able to better choose our carbohydrates based on the ratio of carbohydrates to fiber (in grams per serving) that are listed on the Nutrition Facts label. If the ratio is greater than 10:1 for carbohydrates to fiber, the recommendation is to avoid this food. If the ratio is less than 10:1, it is likely a good choice, and if the ratio is less than 5:1, it is a great choice.

◆ Try to identify the whole grains or oats as the first ingredient on the ingredients list at the bottom of the label for carbohydrate foods. A range of 45 to 65 percent of carbohydrate intake in your total diet is typically recommended. For body composition purposes, much of the current research indicates that the lower end of this spectrum is likely a good thing. This means smart carbohydrate choices (as with all the nutrients) at each meal.

◆ Although there's no gram-per-day recommendation for fat, the U.S. Department of Agriculture provides a general range based on percentage of your total dietary intake, including about 20 to 35 percent of total calories coming from fats. But new research shows that many people successfully eat more fat than this and still improve body composition and health.

◆ A better way to consider fats is by types of fats. Choosing a good mix of polyunsaturated, monounsaturated, and saturated fats is a good idea. Also, limiting omega-6 fatty acids from excessive intake of vegetable oils and premade dressings and increasing intake of omega-3 fatty acids (from fish, nuts, and seeds) is another good idea overall.

◆ As of January 2006, trans fats have been required to be on the Nutrition Facts label. These rarely occur naturally and are considered the *really* bad guys. They're known as lethal because not only do they increase bad cholesterol, but they also decrease good cholesterol and are directly related to heart disease risk. Try to avoid foods high in trans fats.

◆ For fat calories, you need to multiply fat grams by 9, not 4, as you do for both protein and carbohydrates. This means that fat has the highest calorie count per gram of the macronutrients.

◆ Besides the protein, carbohydrates, and fat, also consider the sodium and cholesterol content of foods if you know that you have a negative family or personal disease history with these nutrients. Otherwise, new research indicates far less concern than originally thought.

◆ Also, look at the amount of micronutrients in your food, including vitamins and minerals. A few will be listed on your food label. It is best to aim for 100 percent of the micronutrients in your daily diet from all meals and supplements.

Try This

Read Nutrition Facts labels for sugar content and aim to reduce the amount of added sugars in your overall diet.

Questions to Consider

1. What sources of fat are dominant in your diet?

2. How much added sugar do you get in your typical daily diet?

Nutrient Timing and Frequency

The purpose of this lecture is to discuss the different components of nutrient timing—specifically, pre-exercise, during-exercise, and postexercise nutrition—and to shed some light on which tactics seem to work best for body composition and performance. Keep in mind that although common recommendations exist, nutrition is very individualized. Overall, make sure that you are getting adequate carbohydrates, fats, protein, and micronutrients throughout the day to fuel your lifestyle, and understand that this might differ drastically from person to person. Then, try some timing strategies to see if they work for you.

Nutrient Timing

- Timing when to eat our meals around exercise is important for many reasons. We need energy to fuel our workouts—perhaps multiple bouts in one day—but at the same time, we don't want to eat too much or too close to a training session or we might experience gastrointestinal issues that could make us feel terrible and ruin our workout.

- Nutrient timing is an overarching idea that encompasses a variety of strategies that might be directed toward performance, recovery from strenuous exercise, improving body composition, or a combination of all three.

Pre-Exercise Nutrition

- You need fuel and energy to exercise. Your body needs at least some fuel in the tank to perform optimally. Glycogen, which is the storage form of carbohydrates in the body, is the main fuel source during moderate to vigorous exercise, so it stands to reason that carbohydrates are an important pre-exercise nutrient.

- These energy stores are sometimes the limiting factor in exercise, and running out can be the cause for running out of fuel in many long-distance exercises—essentially, your tank is empty. Thus, it is recommended that consuming carbohydrates prior to exercise (referred to as "carb loading") will fill up the tank. But how much you need depends on what your purpose is and what level of activity you are doing.

- Many leading sports nutritionists instruct IRONMAN athletes—who swim 2.4 miles, bike 112 miles, and then run 26.2 miles—to increase their carbohydrate consumption to about 70 percent of their diet 5 to 7 days before a competition by adding things like oatmeal, rice, pasta, and bread to almost every meal.

- Frankly, the details of optimal pre-exercise nutritional strategies are less important to the average person. That's not to say that pre-exercise nutrition is not important—it certainly is—but simply getting in some good nutrient sources with carbohydrates and protein, ideally 3 to 4 hours before exercise, is all you should concentrate on.

- Be conscious of the total calories that you are taking in and burning during exercise so that you don't end up overeating, adding too much to your total caloric intake, and ultimately hurting your body composition or performance goals.

- Many people prefer to work out in the morning before eating breakfast. If that is you, and you like that, go for it. But if you work out for more than 90 minutes, or at a vigorous intensity, you might consider fueling up a little and see how it makes you feel.

During-Exercise Nutrition

- A common misconception is that you need sugar-filled sports drinks to rehydrate, no matter what type of exercise you are doing. If you are exercising for less than 60 to 90 minutes, all you really need is about a cup of water to keep you hydrated—no extra calories needed.

- If you are participating in long-distance or time-consuming endurance events like marathons, then you certainly need to replenish your body with additional calories during exercise, and sports drinks are a great way to do this.

- For endurance exercise of longer than 60 to 90 minutes, general recommendations for athletes are to take in between 30 and 60 grams of carbohydrates per hour during exercise to extend endurance performance.

- This is a wide range because everybody is different. It is a trial-and-error process to find which fueling strategy works best for you based on what your goals are. If you can only tolerate the lower end of the 30- to 60- gram range, that doesn't mean that you are a worse athlete. Additionally, your stomach—just like your muscles—can be trained to tolerate more.

- This emphasis on eating carbohydrate during exercise becomes even more important if you have not carb loaded, not consumed pre-exercise meals, or have restricted energy intake for weight loss.

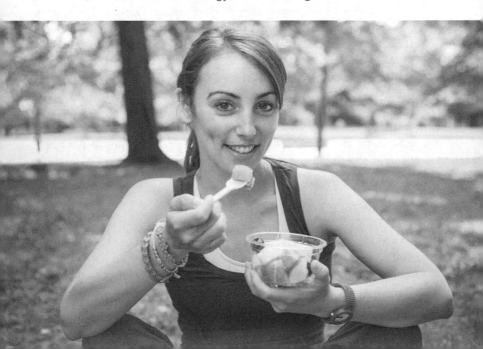

- What type of carbohydrates should you eat before and during exercise? The common recommendation is to eat fast-digesting, or high-glycemic-index, carbohydrates during exercise. These include foods and drinks like sports beverages, premade gels, and whole foods like bread, jelly, and fruit.

- One note of caution is that high-fructose products (such as some sports drinks) and foods (such as a lot of actual fruit) can lead to upset stomach and diarrhea. Most sports drinks have a combination of fructose and glucose, and you need to experiment with them to see what works for you.

- In addition to protein prior to exercise, protein during exercise is important. Decades of research has shown that a carbohydrate-and-protein mix improves performance and lengthens time to exhaustion during endurance exercise when compared to just carbohydrates alone. These studies have all used sports drinks that include carbohydrates and protein.

- The general recommendation for resistance training—because you should be doing a combination of both cardio work and resistance training—is that you include both carbohydrates and protein. The media pushes protein and resistance training so much that many people think that you only need protein during resistance training, but carbohydrates are also important.

- Consuming carbohydrate in combination with protein will provide the most benefits during resistance exercise, and we've seen this in the research for endurance exercise, too. You'll optimize muscle glycogen, encourage better results, and help repair muscles by using a beverage that contains both carbohydrate and protein.

Postexercise Nutrition

- The postexercise period is widely considered the most critical part of nutrient timing. Theoretically, consuming the proper ratio of nutrients immediately following exercise can initiate the rebuilding of damaged muscle tissue and restoration of energy reserves. This might enhance both body composition and exercise performance.

■ This entire concept of consuming nutrients immediately after exercise for maximal gains is often referred to as the "window of opportunity" or your "anabolic window." Generally, this anabolic window is considered to be within 30 and 60 minutes after your workout.

■ The following are some general recommendations for replenishing your fuel stores after exercise.
   ◆ The first issue is your rate of muscle glycogen resynthesis, or how quickly you can restock your stored glucose in your muscles and liver after you depleted them during exercise. Eating carbohydrates within 30 minutes of finishing your exercise seems to result in a greater rate of muscle glycogen resynthesis than if you delay eating carbohydrates by just 2 hours.
   ◆ Some studies have suggested up to 1.5 grams of carbohydrates per kilogram of body weight after a workout. But far less than this amount of carbohydrates will have a beneficial result for glycogen resynthesis.
   ◆ Immediately after exercise, you should aim for a higher-glycemic-index carbohydrate source, such as a bagel, a muffin, pasta, or cereal. Some research shows that a beverage with glucose and fructose might take advantage of certain sugar transporters and allow for the best rate of glycogen resynthesis.
   ◆ The research also shows that adding protein to your carbohydrates after your workout might help further increase glycogen storage and also increase muscle protein synthesis. The ratio of 3 to 4 grams of carbohydrate per 1 gram of protein in the post-workout meal is the general recommendation for these benefits to occur.

■ While there is scientific evidence to support the idea of an anabolic window, it appears as if it is not as important as we originally thought.

■ For athletes who are competing extremely hard and are performing two or more workouts per day, this window is very important to maximize muscle glycogen resynthesis and protein synthesis so that they can begin the recovery process as soon as possible. They need to train or compete within just a few hours.

■ However, for most individuals, while this window still exists, it is not necessary to change your habits to take advantage of it, but doing so might optimize your results. Unless you exercise again within a few hours, you should probably shift your focus more to the total amount of protein and carbohydrate you eat over the course of the day as opposed to hitting that window. For improvements in body composition, it is key to understand your total daily needs.

Meal Frequency

■ The information on how often you should eat, called meal frequency, is all over the place. Some suggest three meals per day while others suggest six, and some even suggest below and above these recommendations.

■ Research suggests that just by increasing protein and eating more frequently, you can improve your body composition, improve satiety, and boost metabolism. But if it's not high in protein, consuming three versus six meals per day doesn't seem to matter.

■ In other words, you can eat several small meals each day or you can eat the traditional three big meals each day, and there's almost no physiological difference. Just decide what you like and what fits your life.

■ Eating frequently might help with optimizing some aspects of performance, body composition, and health, but it is likely overemphasized in many people. Eating frequently might keep you from being over-hungry and gorging at the next meal, but you have to get to know your eating patterns and habits to see if it will work for your lifestyle.

Try This

Try eating six smaller but protein-rich meals per day to see if it works for your lifestyle and goals.

Questions to Consider

1. What will you change with regard to your nutrient timing based on the information from this lecture?

2. Is there a specific food type and timing that is right for you?

Nighttime Eating

For a long time, it was believed that eating late in the night before going to sleep was bad for your health and would automatically make you gain fat. But emerging research has shown that small, protein-type beverages consumed before sleep might have a number of advantages—particularly when paired with a dynamic exercise program. After this lecture, you will have a better understanding of nighttime eating and why many people thought it was off-limits. You will also learn how eating protein at night, particularly before bed, can potentially impact body composition and overall health.

Eating before Bed: Research and Physiology

- We all have a circadian clock, or circadian timing system, that is like an internal clock that regulates our physiology with our daily behaviors and surrounding environment. For many of us, our typical circadian clock keeps us awake and active during the daytime hours and less active during the evening and night hours.

- Our circadian clock adjusts our physiology to coincide with these typical periods of activity and rest throughout the day. Because many of us are less active in the evening and late-night hours, our clock is programmed to slow our internal system down at those times, too.

- But does a less active system at night translate to fat gain if you eat at night? It depends. The food we consume essentially has two fates: It's either stored for later use or burned for energy (oxidation). Because our biological clock slows things down at night, it seems obvious that any food we eat at night will more likely be stored rather than burned during this time. So, this might be strike one against eating at night.

- When you eat carbohydrates, for example, they are broken down into smaller components, like glucose, that enter your blood. In response to the glucose, insulin is secreted from your pancreas to get the glucose into your cells. This effectively lowers blood glucose back to "normal."

- A potential strike two against eating at night is that research shows that for the same amount of glucose, greater amounts of insulin are required to remove it from the blood during the night as compared to the day. More insulin produced means more storage at night.

- If nighttime eating is not done often, there is likely no problem. But if repeated over time, chronically high insulin can lead to desensitization of the insulin receptors and possibly to future problems with glucose control.

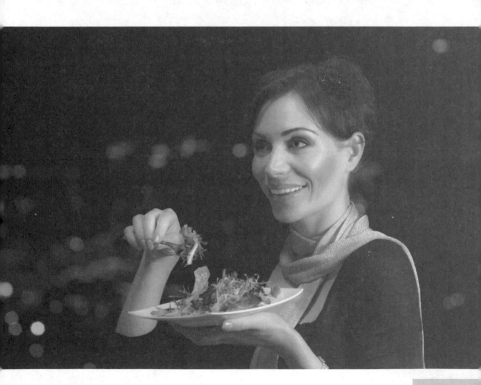

- Research has also shown that the energy cost of digesting and processing your food—that is, the thermic effect of food—decreases at night. That means that if you eat the same exact meal for breakfast as you do for dinner, you'll have lower energy expenditure in the evening.

- We also know that we do not feel as full when we eat food toward the later part of the day, so there's a chance that we'll eat more. In addition, it takes longer for food eaten later in the day to be emptied from the stomach and into the intestines during this time.

- So, our physiology at night favors storage when we eat toward the later part of the day. This might not be ideal for body composition. Based on this information, could nighttime be the wrong time to eat? Is there a wrong time of day for people to eat if they want to maintain or lose fat?

- While some of the research done in this area has been focused on specific groups of people—such as night-shift workers and people with night eating syndrome who ate late at night—and there is also controversy with what defines nighttime eating, the takeaway message is not controversial: If you consume the majority of your food in the evening and night hours as opposed to during the daytime hours and in excess of your energy needs, then you will likely have some unfavorable changes in your body composition.

- But many of us eat our food at various intervals throughout the day and not primarily at one point of the day or another. Also, most people sleep during the night and work during the day.

- So, one way that researchers define nighttime eating, or presleep eating, is simply taking in an additional snack after dinner and before going to bed.

- It might just be a matter of knowing what our best food choices are if we want to eat at night. We know that large portions are not ideal, but what about low-calorie, nutrient-dense options? What about protein?

Consuming Protein before Bed: Active People

- Many athletes and bodybuilders typically consume protein before bed, but are they reaping any benefits? For very active people, the rationale for consuming protein before bed is the belief that it would keep you anabolic overnight and promote muscle growth or repair.

- Remember that "anabolic" means promoting a metabolic environment to stimulate, in this case, muscle building. The idea is that perhaps, over the long term, this continual anabolic state could lead to increases in muscle recovery and performance. Eating protein before bed to keep muscle growth continuing overnight might give you a competitive edge or allow you to recover better.

- Whey protein is a very common supplement used by athletes and everyday gym-goers. However, casein protein, which makes up 80 percent of the protein in milk, has been highlighted as the best to be consumed before sleep due to its slow release from the stomach.

- Casein is found in higher concentrations in foods like cottage cheese and Greek yogurt. The theory is that this allows for prolonged anabolism or, at least, less muscle breakdown overnight while you are sleeping.

- It wasn't until 2012 that research-based evidence on the impact of consuming casein protein before bed was available. Professor Luc Van Loon and his research team in the Netherlands were the first to show us that consuming casein protein before bed increases muscle protein synthesis overnight. The studies demonstrated a few new things: We can digest and absorb protein at night, and we can increase muscle protein synthesis while sleeping.

- In a follow-up study, Professor Van Loon's group was able to show true improvements in body composition when protein was consumed at night during a 12-week resistance exercise program. This shows us that specifically eating protein at night before bed can increase muscle mass in the long term.

- Furthermore, research has shown that providing casein, whey, or carbohydrates within 30 minutes of going to bed led to greater resting energy expenditure (so burning more calories) in physically active men the next morning—compared to the lower resting energy expenditure when the men were given a placebo at night before bed.

- Research has also found that fat burning was better when fit young men drank either a placebo or a casein protein shake compared to when they were given whey protein or carbohydrates.

- This shows that the subjects who drank a placebo, which had no calories, and those who drank about 150 calories of casein protein both responded with a nice fat-oxidation or fat-burning response. This was a better response than provided by drinking whey protein or carbohydrates.

- Taken together, this information tells us that if you are an active individual or athlete, consuming something before bed is better than going to bed on an empty stomach if you want to maximize your calorie-burning potential. It also suggests that casein may be better than whey, because casein seems to increase muscle growth overnight, and may promote a greater fat utilization.

Consuming Protein before Bed: Overweight and Obese People

- Drinking small amounts of protein before bed seems to be beneficial for active people, but what about for overweight and obese people? Remember that the main reason to avoid nighttime eating was because we were told that it would make us store calories rather than burn them—that is, gain fat. But is this the case when you eat specifically after dinner and before sleep *and* you eat only a small portion?

- To answer this, researchers provided a small, low-calorie protein-and-carbohydrate snack (in the form of cereal and milk) to overweight and obese people 90 minutes after dinner. This was opposed to the typical high-calorie, high-fat meals that they were used to eating at night. They did this every day for four weeks.

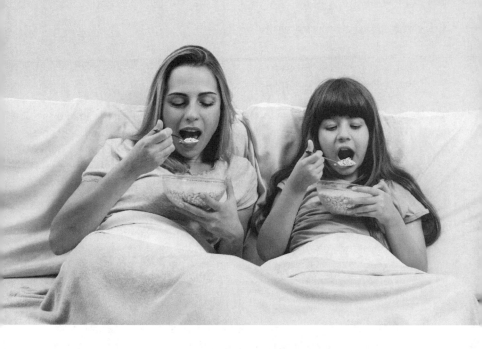

- They found that the people who ate the cereal at night before sleep (which was about 130 calories of food) ended up lowering the total number of calories that they ate all day long on average over the four-week study. This led them to lose body weight in this study.

- Just knowing that you are "allowed" to eat again later in the evening might stop you from taking bigger servings or going for seconds at your other meals. Still, this was the only study to see nighttime feeding in a positive light for people who were not active or fit.

- What would happen if the nighttime snack were a low-calorie protein beverage (of about 150 to 160 calories) instead of the protein plus carb cereal snack?

- Researchers gave one of three beverages—casein protein, whey protein, or a carbohydrate drink—to overweight and obese people within 30 minutes of going to bed and found that the participants felt fuller and had less desire to eat the next morning regardless of what they consumed (protein or carbohydrates).

- Perhaps this was beneficial in terms of reducing total calorie intake the next day, similar to the cereal study. But because the study was only one night long and researchers didn't measure how much food participants ate for breakfast or if they ate less overall as a result of nighttime eating, they don't really know if the presleep snacks had an impact on total calorie intake.

- Unfortunately, researchers also found that all groups, regardless of what they consumed, had higher insulin levels the next morning compared to normal. This was not an ideal finding because obesity is already associated with insulin resistance, or a lowered ability to use the insulin that is produced.

- But the obvious solution to this problem is exercise. Exercise training increases insulin sensitivity, so adding daily exercise over a longer period might stop or reverse this acute insulin resistance associated with eating before bed in overweight and obese people.

- When researchers carried out nighttime feeding of protein or carbohydrates before bed with the subjects for four weeks and added three days per week of exercise training, insulin levels did not change from baseline.

- In addition, the group consuming the casein beverage felt fuller at the end of the four weeks compared to the groups consuming whey and carbohydrates. This study shows a possible advantage to casein protein.

- Furthermore, there were slight decreases in body fat and slight increases in lean mass in all groups, while body weight stayed the same. In other words, there was no change in body weight, but body composition was slightly better.

■ So, it turns out that there might be some real advantages to eating a small protein snack late at night. We also know that increasing protein in your diet is advantageous for body composition over longer studies. This nighttime addition of protein will help increase total protein intake in your day.

Try This

If you are hungry at night before bedtime, try having a small protein beverage or protein food.

Questions to Consider

1. What are some things you tend to eat before bed? What are some alternatives that you can try instead?

2. What are three reasons why you might consider eating a small protein-centric snack before bed?

Evaluating Dietary Supplements

The field of performance nutrition is extremely dynamic. There is new research coming out almost daily that can change the general consensus on any single topic. While there are many performance supplements that show no real benefit, other supplements could be quite beneficial to health, body composition, and performance, as you will learn in this lecture. In fact, some performance supplements have shown safety and efficacy for a long time and have now made their way into the clinical world to alleviate and prevent diseases.

Supplement Facts Panel

- A dietary supplement has a very long definition. Technically, they are defined as a product that is intended to supplement the diet and contains one or more of the following ingredients: a vitamin, mineral, an herb or other botanical, an amino acid that is a concentrate, a metabolite, a constituent, an extract, or a combination of any of these.

- Note that these products are not intended to replace food that is already in your diet.

- There are some differences between a conventional food label with the Nutrition Facts panel and the Supplement Facts panel.

- You'll often see a section with a "proprietary blend" listed. This means that rather than giving specific amounts of specific ingredients, they are bunched together under "proprietary blend," and only a single amount of all ingredients in the blend is listed. This is a list of ingredients that are part of a product formula specific to a particular manufacturer. It is their secret ingredient.

■ The Food and Drug Administration does not require the amount of the ingredients in the proprietary blend formula to be listed, which is where consumers tend to run into trouble with supplements. You don't have to avoid products with a proprietary blend, but be sure to work with a sports nutritionist and your physician to see what will work best for you.

■ If you do see the dose listed—which many quality companies include on their labels already—it's best to be sure that it matches what the research evidence shows actually works for humans.

Fat-Loss Supplements: Caffeine

■ Contrary to what you might think, some fat-burning supplements on the market actually work and are safe. Most of these supplements target fat loss in one of three ways: by increasing the fat you burn for energy, by blocking fat storage in your body, or by controlling your calorie intake by suppressing hunger. However, of all the marketed products, only a few have good research-based evidence.

■ The most common supplement in the fat-burning category is caffeine. In fact, caffeine is the most popularly consumed drug in the world and is found in coffee, tea, soda, and even chocolate.

■ Caffeine is thought to be a weight-loss supplement because it increases resting energy expenditure by 7 to 15 percent in some studies. The active compound of caffeine, called methylxanthine, acts as a heart muscle, skeletal muscle, and central nervous system stimulant. This is why you might get the jitters when you have an extra cup of coffee in the morning.

■ Some people need to be careful because the extra stimulation from caffeine can be too much. But this only needs to really be taken as a precaution if you have a preexisting heart condition or are extremely sensitive to caffeine. As always, check with your doctor regarding your individual health status.

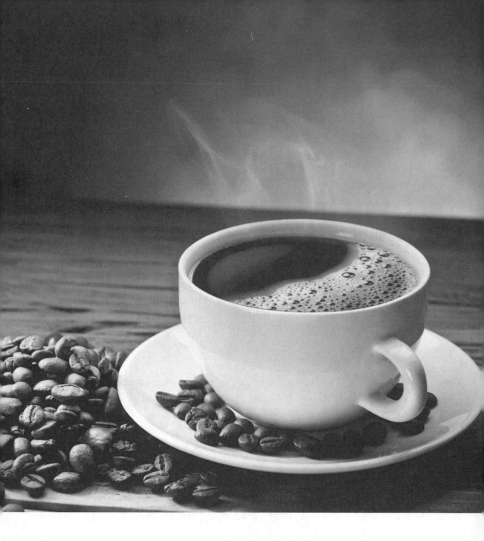

- Most of the studies show that to have a noticeable metabolic-increasing effect, roughly 3 to 6 milligrams of caffeine per kilogram of body mass must be consumed at one time. This equates to about 1 to 2 normal-sized servings, such as 16- to 20-ounce cups of coffee, depending on the strength of the brew.

- If you don't like drinking that much liquid, there are caffeine tablets available on the market that are pretty inexpensive and contain about 200 milligrams per pill. Just keep in mind that an excess of pretty much anything that you put into your body will likely cause problems and could even be deadly.

- You can probably see how this might lead to cost and/or efficacy issues of caffeine. For fat loss, start with many of the other nutrition and exercise factors offered in this course first. Then, if you truly want to try caffeine for fat-loss purposes, it could be useful if done properly.

- It is best to have caffeine 30 to 45 minutes before exercise and/or first thing in the morning before breakfast. For best results, caffeine should be taken on an empty stomach. Consuming it with food, especially carbohydrates, diminishes its effects by lowering plasma caffeine concentrations as well as delaying the time to peak caffeine concentration in your blood.

- Drinking your coffee with little or no additives, such as cream, sugar, or milk, might be most helpful (not to mention lowering your overall calorie intake).

- The downside to caffeine is that the effect of caffeine on weight loss is not the same for everyone. It seems to work best for younger people and for those who are more physically fit.

- Also, if you consume lots of caffeine, it is thought that you become less sensitive to its fat-loss and exercise-performance effects.

- A common concern that people have with caffeine is that it will cause dehydration. However, numerous studies have shown that this is a myth and that there is no evidence to support it.

Fat-Loss Supplements: Green Tea

- Green tea has become increasingly popular in American culture over the past decade, with all kinds of products that contain green tea or green tea extracts. It has been used in Eastern cultures for much longer to increase mental awareness, improve digestion, regulate body temperature, act as an antioxidant, and for its antiobesity and anticancer effects.

- The active ingredient in green tea is called epigallocatechin gallate (EGCG). In some studies, EGCG has been shown to increase energy expenditure by about 4 percent and increase fat burning by 10 percent compared to a placebo.

- Interestingly, when combined with caffeine, there seems to be a synergistic effect between caffeine and EGCG, which in some studies has been shown to ramp up fat burning more than caffeine or EGCG alone.

- But don't run to the supermarket and start buying everything with green tea just yet. To have a beneficial effect, research shows that you need to consume about 750 milligrams, or about 15 cups, per day of EGCG.

- But you don't have to drink all of your EGCG. Many EGCG supplements are found in capsulated form, with about 400 milligrams per pill. Check with your doctor to make sure that your choices are healthy ones.

- Many teas and supplements contain both EGCG and caffeine. But even drinking decaffeinated green tea might improve body composition.

Fat-Loss Supplements: Capsaicin

- Capsaicin is a spice that causes the perceived "hotness" you feel when eating spicy foods. This pungent extract has been shown to increase thermogenesis and energy expenditure.

- The issue with this is that many of these studies use rats and not humans as research subjects. So, you have to be cautious about generalizing results to humans.

- The data for humans is less impressive, but body fat reductions have been reported. The issue is that there is a high rate of weight regain,

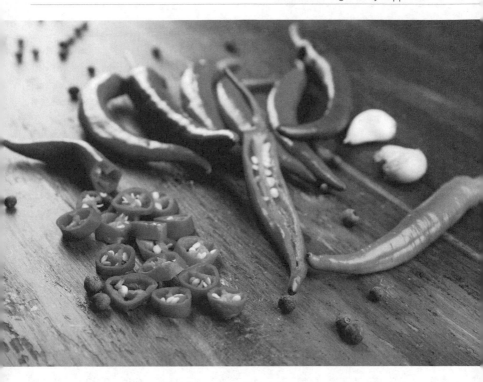

and the participants had trouble sticking to the dosage that is thought to be required for a beneficial effect.

Fat-Loss Supplements: Carnitine

■ Another debatable supplement for fat loss is called carnitine, which is a fat carrier, or gatekeeper, that helps transfer fat into the mitochondria, where it gets oxidized for fuel. Logically, it makes sense to think that if you increase the amount of carnitine, then you could get more fat into the right place to burn for energy.

■ Unfortunately, that is not the case in 99 percent of the research on this topic. Until more long-term studies are completed, it doesn't appear to be worth it.

Muscle-Gain Supplements: Creatine

- The biggest player in the category of supplements that are thought to increase your muscle mass is creatine, or creatine monohydrate. Creatine is one the most popular supplements ever produced and the most thoroughly researched of any supplement.

- We produce creatine naturally in the liver and kidneys. It is stored either as free creatine or bound to a phosphate in skeletal muscle. Naturally, the creatine phosphate energy system is used to provide energy for maximal-intensity, short-duration exercise. Creatine supplies a phosphate to adenosine diphosphate to create adenosine triphosphate, or ATP—the energy we need to do everything.

- As a supplement, creatine is often used to help build muscle, improve strength and power, and increase anaerobic, short-duration exercise (i.e., power lifting or sprinting). The standard serving of creatine is 5 grams, which is equal to the amount of creatine in about 2.5 pounds of raw meat. So, it is much easier to take a small scoop of creatine versus eating an entire plate of steak.

- There are several forms of creatine on the market, but the one that has the most research support and effectiveness is creatine monohydrate. Several hundred peer-reviewed research studies have evaluated this form, and more than 70 percent of these studies show a significant improvement in exercise capacity and increases in muscle mass.

- Most experts attribute the beneficial changes to body composition and performance from creatine to the improved ability to do more quality work during exercise. But research also shows some improvements to actual cellular processes for muscle gain, too.

- And due to the repeatable success of creatine use for improving both body composition and performance, creatine is now being studied and used with great interest for use with clinical populations and in disease prevention.

- Creatine has now been shown to improve muscle mass and outcomes in people with muscular dystrophy, leukemia, traumatic brain injury, and infants born with errors in normal metabolic function.

- A common myth is that creatine is a steroid and will damage your kidneys. Creatine is not a steroid; it is simply the combination of three amino acids. The research shows that creatine is safe and effective among young and old, male and female, and healthy and diseased populations. In the absence of any preexisting conditions, such as kidney disease, creatine is a supplement that has consistently been shown to be beneficial.

- The most common side effect reported is weight gain. However, this is probably the type that you want, because creatine increases muscle mass. Also note that some cases of gastrointestinal upset have been noted in the literature. The most common dose is 5 grams per day (about 1 tablespoon).

Muscle-Gain Supplements: Beta-Alanine

- Another supplement that might help with muscle mass and performance is called beta-alanine, which has been shown to improve performance and exercise capacity as well as permit greater intensity and volume of exercise training.

- Beta-alanine, which is an amino acid made in the liver, combines with another amino acid called histidine to form a new protein molecule called carnosine in the muscle. Carnosine then acts to buffer, or soak up, the acidity, or hydrogen ions, that is created during very difficult exercise.

- When accumulated, hydrogen ions cause muscle pain and fatigue, so if the hydrogen ions are controlled, theoretically, you could exercise longer and/or at a higher intensity. And higher-intensity exercise for longer should help improve body composition.

- Many studies support the use of beta-alanine to increase performance and body composition in both men and women. About 3 to 6 grams per day for 4 weeks can increase intramuscular carnosine and improve performance. Typically, this dose should be split up throughout the day for best results.

- One side effect to note is that beta-alanine is often associated with a tingling feeling or numbness in the extremities called paresthesia. It is temporary but annoying. And not all people have this feeling, but it is reported in many of the research studies. As a result, some companies have made extended-release capsules to allow a slow release of beta-alanine, which can help reduce or diminish any of the paresthesia effects.

Try This

Try adding 5 grams per day of creatine monohydrate to your daily routine.

Questions to Consider

1. What supplements do you already take? Are there any supplements hidden in common foods or beverages that you consume?

2. What myths have been busted based on the new information you've learned from this lecture? What supplements do you think you would be willing to try after learning what you learned in this lecture?

Energy Balance and Weight Control

This lecture will cover the topic of energy balance and weight control. You will learn about the major components of food and exercise that might shift your energy balance to favor weight loss or weight gain. The point is to expand your understanding of how energy balance contributes to changes in body composition and health. You will also learn what situations impact your calorie burn and the common ways that you might easily fall into a positive energy balance without even knowing it.

Food Intake and Energy Expenditure

- Most people don't track food intake or bother to read labels or weigh food items. This might not be a practical way to live your life, but it can be useful for some people, even if you just periodically check your calorie intake to keep yourself on track.

- Knowing the relationship between your food intake and energy expenditure can be extremely helpful for figuring out if you will lose weight, maintain weight, or gain weight. The quality of your food choices makes a big difference in weight loss and weight gain goals, but at some point, knowing your routine calorie intake and expenditure is a good idea, too, and often a great place to start if you want to be more active in managing your body composition.

- Many of our official dietary recommendations are based on the calorie content of foods. While this intention was good, it puts certain high-calorie but nutrient-dense foods like nuts, seeds, and eggs into a high-caution list, simply because the calorie content is high.

- We know now that these foods are actually beneficial for weight loss and prevention of weight gain when added to the diet. But when considering only the calorie content, they mistakenly seem like a bad choice.

■ Even more interesting is that foods like whole eggs are often considered in the same category of "eat sparingly" as cookies and cakes. But eggs and cookies/cake have very different impacts physiologically.

■ Nevertheless, even if certain foods might be associated with weight loss or gain, calories ultimately do matter, to some extent, in your weight-management success.

■ The energy balance equation is used with regard to body weight control. Energy balance simply means that the energy that you expend from normal daily energy needs (such as breathing, staying awake, digestion and absorption, and physical activity) or extra activity (such as exercise) is matched or balanced by the energy that you take in from foods and beverages.

■ There are three basic conditions to be aware of with the energy balance equation: energy balance, where the food calories that you take in match the calories that you expend or burn; positive energy balance, where you eat more calories than expended (or more in than out); and negative energy balance, where more energy is expended than consumed (or more out than in).

■ Theoretically, if you are in energy balance, you will not lose or gain any weight. In a positive energy balance, you will gain weight. In a negative energy balance, you will lose weight.

■ Regardless of whether you're in a positive or negative energy balance, there are numerous changes that occur to your body—cellularly, metabolically, and hormonally—to facilitate weight gain or loss.

■ When we think about energy balance, we need to pay attention to how many calories we need to eat and drink to begin losing weight (or perhaps gaining weight). This is not considering the quality of calories, though.

Energy In

- How many calories do you need to cut from your diet, or what deficit do you need to create, to lose weight? How many calories will it take to lose just one pound?

- For years, textbooks and experts have asserted that one pound of fat is equivalent to 3,500 calories. So, if you aim for a reduction in one pound of fat per week by modifying your diet alone (not considering exercise), then you would simply eat 500 fewer calories per day for one week.

- If you eat 500 fewer calories per day and lose one pound per week, why not up this to a reduction of 1,000 calories per day or more from your typical diet and lose 2 or 3 pounds per week? The "more is better" mantra does not always suit us well with diet or exercise.

- If your energy deficit is more than about 1,000 calories per day, it is generally not well tolerated. This is due to many factors, but primarily when you drop your calories by too much, you will also lose muscle—which you do not want.

- Too great a calorie deficit also runs a greater risk of missing out on key nutrients, such as vitamins and minerals, and you would likely see your energy levels drop and your fatigue increase—not to mention, you'll probably feel hungry.

- One myth that has come about from this 3,500-calorie rule is that weight will simply continue to drop at the same rate—otherwise known as a linear model of weight loss. But it turns out that this rule actually greatly overestimates weight loss, meaning that 3,500 calories might translate to less than one pound of weight loss.

- So, an update was made, and the new model for weight loss is called the thermodynamic model, or simply the dynamic model, of weight loss and takes into consideration your baseline body composition, age, height, sex, and degree of calorie restriction. This results in a curvilinear pattern of weight loss over time rather than the traditional linear model of weight loss and is much more accurate in actual trends for weight loss.

Counting Calories

- Food contains energy that has the potential to be converted into useful work once metabolized, or broken down, by your body. That energy is measured in units called calories. So, what is a calorie, and how do we know how many calories are in each food we choose to eat?

- Technically, a calorie is a unit of heat measurement defined as the amount of energy required to raise the temperature of one kilogram of water by one degree Celsius. By using this definition, you are actually describing a kilocalorie, which is the type of calorie that you see on nutrient labels.

- In reality, calories are sort of made up. You don't really eat calories; you eat different kinds of food with different amounts of nutrients in them. However, we give foods a calorie count by burning them in a bomb calorimeter and measuring how much heat is given off.

- Each gram of carbohydrate equals 4 calories. A gram of protein also equals 4 calories, and a gram of fat equals 9 calories. When you burn 1 gram of carbohydrate, 4.18 calories are released. When you burn 1 gram of protein, 5.65 calories are released, and when you burn 1 gram of fat, 9.44 calories are released.

- These numbers can vary by the type of carbohydrate, protein, and fat that you burn, as well. And these numbers are slightly different than the 4, 4, 9 that are commonly taught in nutrition and exercise science classes.

- This is because the digestion and absorption rates of nutrients are less than 100 percent in most foods. This results in a reduced energy intake than when measured by direct calorimetry in a bomb calorimeter.

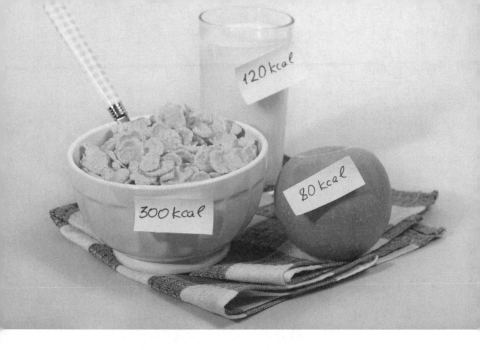

- Many factors impact how many calories you actually can use in your body. Some of these might be how the food is grown, such as the soil conditions, what the animal's diet contained, and how ripe the food was when harvested. Even how you cook or prepare the meal makes a difference.

- In general, the macronutrient with the highest coefficient of digestibility is carbohydrates at 97 percent, followed by fats at 95 percent and proteins at 92 percent. There can also be variation within a food category.

- So, the process of determining the calories in foods is probably more extensive than you imagined. It might also be a shock to see how inexact the process is. In fact, the calories listed on food labels are really just approximations because the data from the bomb calorimeter has a degree of variability.

Energy Out

■ Just as we can measure the calories contained in certain foods, we have ways to scientifically measure the energy that you expend each day. Direct calorimetry is the most accurate way to measure your energy expenditure, but it is very expensive and highly impractical. You don't actually go into a bomb calorimeter and ignite, but the process is similar in many ways.

■ Indirect calorimetry, which measures within ± 1 percent of the direct method, is more often used in lab settings. Indirect calorimetry measures your breath—specifically the oxygen that you use and the carbon dioxide that you exhale.

■ On average, about 5 calories are burned for every 1 liter of oxygen that you consume. Using this fact as well as indirect calorimetry, we can calculate how many calories you are burning and from which macronutrient.

■ This is done by determining the respiratory exchange ratio, which is calculated by dividing the amount of carbon dioxide produced or exhaled by the amount of oxygen that you consume or inhale. Values range between 0.7 and 1. Even though things like hyperventilation or excessive acid buffering in the cells can skew this ratio a bit, it does give an excellent estimation of fuel use.

■ By understanding how much of what type of fuel you are burning for energy, you have a good idea of energy expenditure, which you need with your calorie intake to calculate your overall energy balance and primary nutrient needs for your lifestyle. Even better, you will also have a huge advantage from knowing how the foods you eat impact this balance and, ultimately, why and how eating and exercising contribute to your body composition.

■ There are also many very good metabolic equations—such as Harris-Benedict equation and the Cunningham equation—that have been developed to estimate energy expenditure. These equations are based on many things, such as age, gender, height, weight, and daily activity levels. These formulas are an excellent place to start and give a practical estimate when used properly.

■ It is important to remember that these equations are only estimations. Metabolism is constantly changing based on the needs of the individual, so it is important to reevaluate a person's nutrition plan based on performance, body weight, and body composition over time.

Total Daily Energy Expenditure

■ Four components contribute to your total daily energy expenditure, or all of the calories that you burn in a day.

◆ Resting metabolic rate, which is the energy required to maintain the systems of your body at rest.

◆ Thermic effect of food, which is the amount of energy required to digest the food you eat.

◆ Thermic effect of activity, which is the energy expended doing active things, such as working around the house or doing structured exercise.

◆ Non-exercise activity thermogenesis, which includes unplanned activity, such as tapping your feet or bouncing your knees.

■ Of the components of our total daily energy expenditure, by far the largest is your resting metabolic rate. About 60 to 80 percent of the oxygen you consume and calories you burn goes to just keeping you alive at rest.

■ Many factors influence resting metabolic rate, including age, sex, genetics, energy intake (whether fasting or fed), body size, lean body mass, body temperature or climate, caffeine or nicotine consumption, and exercise. Obviously, there are some uncontrollable characteristics that play a part in determining it.

■ Huge meals with high calorie counts have a larger thermic effect of food. Protein-rich foods also have the greatest effect on increasing calorie burn, because they are the most difficult to digest and absorb—which is one reason that added protein in the diet can be helpful for body composition.

- The amount of exercise and activity you do will determine how much of a role the thermic effect of activity and non-exercise activity thermogenesis play into your overall energy expenditure.

Try This

Calculate your resting metabolic rate to have an idea about your daily caloric needs.

Questions to Consider

1. What sources of carbohydrate in your diet would be best for optimizing your body composition?

2. How much added sugar do you think you consume in your typical daily diet?

The Caloric Cost of Exercise

This lecture will take a closer look at the ways we can expend energy and how we might use that information in our efforts to strengthen or alter our body composition. There are many different types of exercise that can help you reach your goals—from small adjustments, such as taking the stairs at work, walking around more, and perhaps getting a standup desk if you have a desk job, to full-blown structured exercise plans. As you will learn, the body needs a combination of proper fueling and exercise to optimize its potential.

The Caloric Cost of Exercise

- If you want to manipulate your body composition, it is important to know the quality of your calories, how many calories you are eating and drinking, and how many calories you are expending.

- Various types of exercises demand varying amounts of energy—walking versus running, for example—and these energy demands are measured scientifically through metabolic testing, which measures the amount of oxygen you take in during an activity. The more strenuous or intense the activity is, the greater the oxygen consumption.

- We have all kinds of technology that estimate calories burned, but not long ago, the caloric cost of exercise was traditionally measured in metabolic equivalents (mets). You might have seen the term "mets" on the exercise equipment in your home or at the local gym. It is simply another way to assess or quantify the intensity level of your exercise.

- One metabolic equivalent is equal to the oxygen consumption of your body at rest, or 3.5 milliliters per kilogram of body weight per minute. When measuring mets, everything is compared to the cost of energy at rest. The more strenuous the exercise, the higher the met value will be—that is, the higher the caloric expenditure will be in relation to resting.

- Using mets as a measure of your exercise intensity might seem strange, but if you are trying to determine the number of calories you burn when you are exercising—in other words, your caloric cost of exercise—then a great estimate is to simply multiply the met value by your body weight in kilograms.

- Calories are essential; don't treat them as the enemy. Food is fuel. Fuel your body properly for optimal body composition and performance in any aspect of your life—mental or physical.

- For most of us, our main energy source during exercise comes in the form of muscle glycogen. Your body has plenty of fuel to perform most forms of exercise—generally about two hours of moderate- to high-intensity exercise.

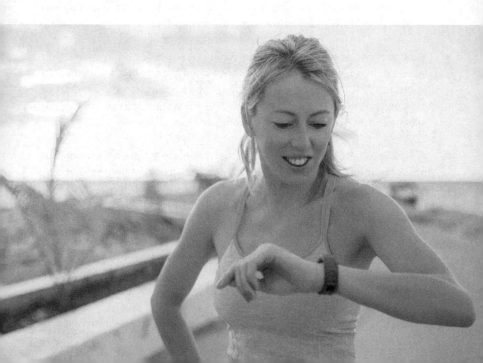

- But sometimes we do run out, which is part of the reason you see athletes collapse from time to time. Their bodies have run out of the ability to access and utilize fuel. They might have the mental fortitude to continue, but the body's systems begin to shut down.

- The body is remarkable at properly operating all of its intricate systems most of the time—from muscles to enzymes to atoms—in complete unison. But it requires good-quality fuel.

Exercise and Your Metabolism

- Exercise increases your caloric expenditure above resting levels, or your resting metabolic rate (RMR), based on how long and intensely you exercise. But does this increase in metabolism last after you finish exercising? In other words, does this increase in caloric expenditure help you burn more calories throughout the day?

- Research has shown that your energy expenditure does remain elevated after cessation of exercise. But it is important to note that the amount of elevation in metabolism is dependent primarily on the intensity of the exercise and, to a lesser degree, the duration of your exercise. In other words, what you do during exercise makes a difference in your RMR.

- Pretty much the same concept applies to lifting weights. Plenty of research has shown that vigorous weight training can increase your metabolic rate for hours after exercise. However, the average person who takes long breaks between sets will likely not see a large enough elevation to play a significant role on total daily energy expenditure.

- You might have heard, too, that exercise increases your RMR all day long—meaning 24 hours or more. There has been quite a bit of research showing that the combination of high exercise energy expenditure and high energy intake in endurance-trained people can elevate RMR for a short period of time (from a few hours all the way up to about 24 hours), but not permanently.

- However, there doesn't seem to be substantial evidence that this elevated RMR will occur at all with normal, recreationally active people—although some research has shown benefits in the elderly.

- The effect of weight training on RMR is interesting. Weight training might play a large role in total daily energy expenditure—but the caveat is that it's not likely to dramatically increase your RMR, or postexercise energy expenditure, outside of the exercise itself.

- How does high-intensity interval training (HIIT) compare to endurance training in burning calories and raising your RMR?

- If you are trying to lose weight and improve body composition through exercise, it's likely that you have been told to do aerobic exercise because it is thought to increase both cardiorespiratory fitness and to help lose weight and fat.

- Most aerobic exercise interventions consist of moderate-intensity steady-state exercise for about 30 to 40 minutes for 3 to 4 days per week over a 4- to 6-month period. Unfortunately, research on these kinds of exercise programs, more often than not, have shown only a minimal fat loss. In contrast, a lot of the research shows that HIIT exercise results in significant fat loss.

- This might sound counterintuitive because you know that higher-intensity exercise burns more carbohydrates, while lower-intensity exercise burns more fat. However, the key to body fat manipulation is all about the total number of calories burned.

- Luckily, some research has directly compared traditional aerobic exercise to HIIT. One study showed that young women in a group who did HIIT lost 2.5 kilograms, or about 5.5 pounds, more fat over the course of a 15-week exercise plan than did the aerobic group—in about half of the exercise time. In other words, higher-intensity exercise might be much more time efficient for weight loss and improvement in body composition.

- The caloric cost of this type of exercise will benefit us all. In fact, much of the research regarding HIIT shows that individuals can exercise for a shorter duration but still lose more fat, gain more muscle, and thus improve body composition and health to a greater degree than they can with a traditional aerobic program.

Non-Exercise Calorie Burn

- What about caloric expenditure when you're not exercising? What you do the rest of your day can also make a big difference in your physical activity levels and body composition.

- A common misperception is that only physical activity or exercise—such as running, biking, walking, or lifting weights—is needed to get any sort of health benefit. However, just as snacking on the wrong things throughout the day can make you gain weight, small acts of physical activity throughout the day can make you healthier and even improve body composition.

- Very simple things—such as taking the stairs rather than taking the escalator or elevator—can improve your health over the course of time by adding to the total caloric expenditure of the day.

- Not only does taking the stairs improve leg strength and cardiovascular fitness, but research has shown that the average person will burn just more than 1 calorie per stair they climb, or about 15 calories for every flight of stairs. This caloric expenditure is based on a 150- to 160-pound person, so a lighter person will burn fewer calories and a heavier person will burn more.

- In addition, research has shown that walking down stairs burns about one-third the number of calories as climbing stairs—so about 5 calories per flight descended, making a total of 20 calories per time you go up and down a flight of stairs. Furthermore, more often than not, you will actually save time taking the stairs.

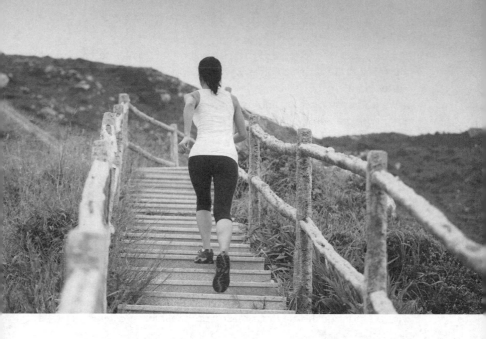

- Over the course of a month or a year, these calories add up and can really improve your health and help you improve your body composition, without even working out. Simple daily habits can consciously be altered to improve your health.

- You might be pretty sedentary if you are sitting down at work for too long, even if you exercise most days of the week for a certain amount of time. In a typical workweek, people spend on average six hours per day sitting at their desks.

- If this is the case for you, consider buying a standup desk for your office. Changing to a standing desk can reduce your risk of obesity, type 2 diabetes, cardiovascular disease, cancer, and overall mortality.

- Your heart rate naturally increases as you change from lying down to sitting to standing, and the difference from sitting to standing is approximately 5 to 10 beats per minute, which equates to 0.35 to 0.7 calories per minute.

■ While this doesn't sound like much, it adds up to somewhere between 25 and 50 calories per hour for a simple change. Given that the average person spends 5 hours and 41 minutes per day sitting at a desk, simply standing instead of sitting could burn almost 285 calories.

■ If you stand, you'll probably want to start standing for short periods and work up to longer durations. And make sure that you keep shifting around while you stand.

■ Improved health and body composition do not happen overnight. Changing habits over the long term are what really make the difference, and small changes as well as larger ones matter.

Try This

Pick a new form of activity and include it at least once per week in your weekly routine.

Questions to Consider

1. How can you adapt your daily routine to add simple ways of increasing your energy expenditure? Can you take the stairs? Can you add a short walk or exercise every hour at work?

2. What is the major determining factor for keeping your metabolism high after a workout?

Exercise for Fat Loss

To lose fat and gain muscle at the same time, you must understand which types of exercise will promote fat loss and which types of exercise will promote muscle gain, and how they can be used in conjunction with each other to achieve the best of both worlds. This lecture will focus on exercise—specifically, aerobic exercise and resistance exercise—to increase fat loss. You will examine these types of exercise and learn the science behind how fat loss works.

Aerobic Exercise versus Resistance Exercise

- There are two major categories of exercise: aerobic exercise (such as walking, running, swimming, or cycling) and resistance exercise (such as lifting weights or doing body-weight strength movements).

- Aerobic exercise is repetitive and relies on the continuous activation of the heart and lungs, often called cardiovascular, or cardiorespiratory, exercise. Most people think that aerobic exercise is the key to fat loss.

- Resistance exercise is less continuous and involves moving or lifting objects with forceful muscle contractions. Resistance exercise is typically related to gains in muscle mass, but plenty of evidence shows that it is actually excellent for fat loss and body composition improvements.

- Most major governing bodies that provide exercise recommendations, such as the American College of Sports Medicine, suggest using both aerobic and resistance exercise. This should provide benefits for both improving health and body composition. A combination of exercise types is also a good idea for fat loss.

Aerobic Exercise: Mode

- There are several factors we can manipulate to maximize fat loss when it comes to aerobic exercise.
  - ◆ The mode, or type, of exercise.
  - ◆ The duration of the exercise.
  - ◆ The intensity of the exercise.
  - ◆ The frequency of exercise, or how often you work out.

- In general, keep in mind that something is better than nothing. The more physical work we do, the more calories we burn, and the greater chance for our total calorie deficit to help with fat loss. But there are certain choices we can make to maximize our aerobic exercise, specifically for the greatest fat loss for a given time spent exercising. This includes altering mode, duration, intensity, and frequency of exercise.

- Much of the mode of aerobic exercise comes down to your personal preferences.
  - ◆ What do you enjoy doing?
  - ◆ What is your accessibility to certain equipment, such as a bike or a pool?
  - ◆ What time of year is it? Is it snowy or really hot?
  - ◆ What is your injury history? Certain activities might be less stressful to achy joints or problem areas.

- The more movement you do, the better. So, if you run versus just sit on a recumbent bike, for the same amount of time, you will probably have more effective fat loss with running because you are using both your upper and lower body during exercise. With more muscles being worked, more overall energy is usually expended.

- Swimming requires both upper- and lower-body muscle groups. But it seems that for a given intensity, swimming will expend fewer calories than either running or cycling. It is thought that the reduced energy expenditure for equally intense swimming exercise might be related to a

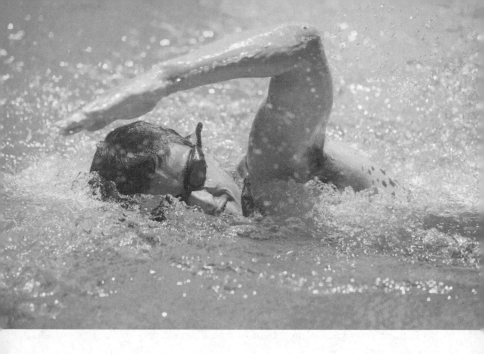

lower heart rate during swimming compared to running or cycling, even when it feels like you are working out at the same effort.

- The primary reason for this is your body position during each exercise. In a more upright exercise, such as running or biking, the heart must work to a larger extent against gravity to return blood to the heart. Swimming, however, requires you to lie flat. In this position, blood travels back to the heart quite easily. This requires less work for the heart and a lower heart rate.

- Swimming in cool water might also increase your total calorie burn. This is because you not only have to work hard just to swim, but you also have to keep your body temperature within a normal range. This concept also stands for running or cycling outside in the cold.

- Aerobic classes, such as step or dance, are not a bad idea, especially if they make exercise more enjoyable for you. However, it is often more difficult to regulate intensity in these types of classes and it also might be a less continuous form of exercise than some other choices, with small breaks given occasionally.

▪ In general, running might actually be the most optimal aerobic exercise type for fat loss specifically. However, if you loathe running or cannot run due to musculoskeletal limitations or injuries, every other form of movement is good and can result in significant improvements in your body composition when paired with solid nutritional choices and lifestyle habits.

Aerobic Exercise: Duration and Intensity

▪ The length of time you exercise and the number of calories you burn are directly and linearly related. The longer you work, the more calories you burn.

▪ If you want the body composition changes that two hours of exercise would give you but you only have 45 minutes to spare in a day, you can burn the same number of calories in 45 minutes that you could over two hours by changing one thing about the way you exercise: the intensity of your exercise.

▪ Intensity is king when it comes to fat loss. Intensity is a measure of how hard you are working. This can be measured by how you feel or quantified by heart rate, exercise speed, or incline.

▪ A major misconception is the idea that low-intensity exercise is better for fat loss. Low-intensity exercise is often called the "fat burn zone." You can actually lose a whole lot of fat by exercising for far less time per day, but you must work out very hard.

▪ This is where high-intensity interval training (HIIT) enters the picture: You simply intermix rest periods with very high-intensity work. So, you might run fast for 1 minute and then "recover" at a slow jog pace for 1 minute and repeat this for 20 minutes.

- High-intensity exercise will burn more fuel than low-intensity exercise. When we exercise at higher intensities, we will burn more carbohydrates for energy, and when we exercise at lower intensities, we will burn more fat for energy. However, using fat for fuel during exercise will not result in the greatest overall losses to total body fat over time. So, the fat burn zone might not be named appropriately, and it's misleading.

- With a high-intensity workout, you will burn energy during and after the exercise, too. But just how much will you burn is dependent on, most importantly, how hard you exercise and somewhat on how long you exercise.

- If your main reason not to exercise is your time, then this technique of going very hard but for a short time eliminates that excuse. Try warming up with a few minutes of walking and things like jumping jacks, lunges, or body-weight squats, and then break your workout session into segments of high-intensity efforts and easy recovery.

- You can find access to a number of interval or HIIT workouts online, in training books, or from a coach. Some interval workouts go by minutes, some go by distance, and some just go by how you feel. But the goal is always to work hard during the active, or work, phase and then recover for a period of time before the next active phase.

- As you become more fit, you can extend the "hard" work phase and decrease the recovery time. A reasonable place to start could be 30 seconds of very hard work followed by 1 minute of easy recovery.

- You might even find interval exercise to be more enjoyable, because it breaks down your workout into segments and makes the time go by more quickly.

- Research shows that interval training results in a greater overall adherence to exercise and might be more enjoyable than continuous lower-intensity exercise. Research also shows that interval training combined with resistance training is incredibly effective for reducing

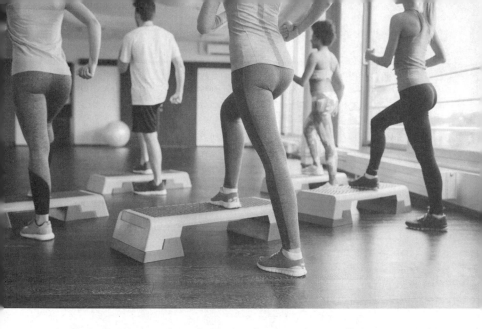

body fat levels. HIIT has also been shown to be as effective, or maybe even more effective, at improving heart health than low-intensity exercise that burned the same number of calories.

- A high level of activity is very difficult, so you really shouldn't do it every day. It is best to mix in days of HIIT and days of slow- to moderate-intensity aerobic exercise. This should help maximize fat loss and keep you from getting hurt.

- And start with an amount of time that you can fit into your schedule. We have shown great results with HIIT for just 20 to 30 minutes! Essentially, you can start with very little exercise and have a great response for improving your body composition.

Aerobic Exercise: Frequency

- Frequency refers to the number of times you exercise per week. For general health, you should exercise three to five days per week, according to the American College of Sports Medicine guidelines.

- For fat loss, it's best to incorporate multiple types of exercise, such as aerobic, HIIT, and resistance. But for aerobic endurance exercise, there are a few ways to get the most possible fat loss from your workouts.
  - Move lots of muscles.
  - Choose higher-intensity exercise through interval training rather than low-intensity exercise, even when the caloric cost is the same.
  - Exercise longer rather than shorter when comparing exercises of the same intensity.
  - Exercise at least five days per week to see the most improvement.

- If you are feeling overwhelmed, don't worry. It is best to only make one change at a time. For example, try to change up your exercise in one small way today that is practical for you. Then, little by little, you can incorporate more of these options to maximize fat loss. It is not a good idea to change everything at once—in fact, that is a sure way to failure.

Resistance Training

- A number of research studies have demonstrated that combining HIIT and resistance training is most effective for fat loss and improving body composition. Resistance training is a very powerful tool for changing body composition.

- With only aerobic exercise, it is far easier to change your overall size but much more difficult to alter the way it looks physically. You can change from a "big pear" shape to a "small pear" shape, but you need to add resistance exercise if you want to add lean muscle and change the way you look.

- Adding lean mass from resistance training is important for fat loss specifically. The addition of resistance training to your activity might kill two or three birds with one stone.
  - It will add lean muscle mass, which is metabolically active. This means that it uses a few more calories than other tissues and contributes to your total daily caloric output.
  - Resistance training increases lipolysis, or fat mobilization.

◆ Resistance training also increases excess postexercise oxygen consumption (EPOC), just like aerobic exercise, but maybe even more.

■ Combining the fat-burning effects of aerobic and resistance exercise seems to offer the maximal benefits for fat loss. The combination also looks to be more favorable than aerobic exercise alone in combating certain types of chronic disease, including muscle wasting, osteoporosis, and perhaps even type 2 diabetes.

Try This

Replace one of your longer, slower exercise sessions with short, high-intensity intervals each week.

Questions to Consider

1. What exercise barriers to losing fat do you see in your lifestyle?

2. Where in your week can you fit in aerobic and resistance exercise?

Exercise for Healthy Muscle Mass

This lecture will tackle one of the most widely discussed, and often misguided, topics of interest in this field: muscle. You will learn why you want to increase muscle mass and how to do it, as well as how to properly maintain it and the health benefits of doing so, especially as you age. You will also learn about the type, volume, frequency, and intensity of exercises that induce muscle growth, and you will explore some of the new schools of training that are becoming increasingly popular.

Resistance Training and Aging

- As we age, a phenomenon called sarcopenia occurs, which is the natural, progressive loss of muscle mass as we grow older. Studies have shown that between the ages of 40 and 50, we can lose more than 8 percent of our muscle mass, and that can accelerate to more than 15 percent per decade after the age of 75 if measures are not taken to prevent it. Fortunately, there is a lot we can do to slow down this process.

- Most people think that aging alone causes us to lose muscle. But now research is clearly showing that it is more the lack of physical activity that is the major player here. Long-term exercise training can aid in preserving muscle mass. It might also prevent increases in body fat as we age.

- Resistance training adds muscle, too—if you specifically plan your program with muscle gain as one of your goals. Data show that as you age, the importance of strength is critical. In fact, just being stronger in your chest and legs is associated with the least risk of premature death.

- Resistance training must be included in your exercise program, and there might be some nutritional supplements that can help even more with improving body composition and performance.

Finding a Personal Trainer

- What specifically should you do to increase your muscle mass? As with most well-designed exercise training programs, you should have a balance between strength and endurance training (with your ultimate goal the key factor in how much or little of each you do). You know the difference between low-intensity/steady-state aerobic exercise and HIIT training and the benefits of both.

- Considering that most of the best athletes hire a coach or trainer, you might want to consider hiring a personal trainer, too. If you are an elite athlete or if you are new to exercise, hiring a personal trainer or coach is a great way to start or work on a new goal or to prepare for a race or competition. This way, you can try new exercises, avoid injury, learn about your exercise and lifting options, and figure out how to lift safely while also working around past injuries.

- When choosing a personal trainer, the first step is to figure out if you want to work out in a gym setting or have a personal trainer come to your house. Both are great options, and you just need to find what suits your lifestyle, personality, goals, and budget.

- Some trainers offer gentle encouragement, and others are "in your face" to try and motivate you. The last thing you want is someone giving mild-mannered instruction when you know that does nothing to motivate you. And, likewise, you don't want a drill sergeant type if you respond best to gentle but persistent encouragement.

- Personal trainers should also be held to some educational and certification standards. Don't be shy about directly asking them about these things. Then, take note—because there are some so-called certifications that you can get with an hour of free time and Internet

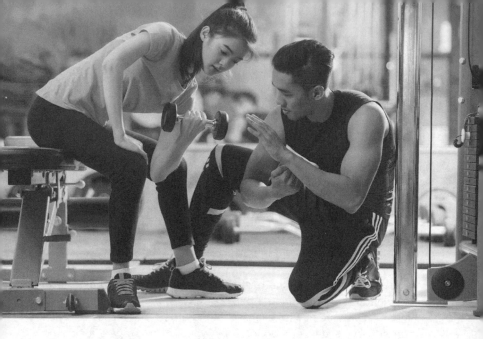

access. Some of the top certifications require a bachelor's degree before you can even sit to take the exams.

- Just like any skilled profession, referrals will help you decide, too. Trainers should be able to provide you with some contact information for people they have trained with similar goals.

- Also ask about how they measure your success and how they progress clients. Observe them with another client and see how they behave. Does the trainer ignore the client and mindlessly count reps while texting or talking on the phone? Do not hire this type of trainer. Training sessions should be about you, your safety, and your goals.

- If you have any special needs (for example, surgeries, sore joints, or known muscle imbalances), be sure to ask if the trainer has credentials and experience with these situations. You also want to ask about the payment structure and make sure that suits your needs. In the end, a good trainer should be extremely transparent so that the client-trainer relationship works for everyone.

- It's not as scary as it sounds once you ask the right questions. Realize, too, that you don't need a personal trainer forever. It is a great tool to have, but if you just want some instruction from time to time, personal trainers can assist with that, too.

Developing an Exercise Program

- With or without a trainer, you need to develop an exercise program. The most important thing to keep in mind is that every program should be individualized. Everyone's goals are different, and that is extremely important to consider.

- A person new to exercise will have a different plan than an elite collegiate athlete or a power lifter. And as research into the science and application of sports science grows, new insights will emerge.

- The American College of Sports Medicine (ACSM) guidelines take into account the recommendations of experts across many disciplines, such as exercise science, physiology, athletic training, and medicine. The ACSM recommends lifting weights a minimum of two to three days per week if you use a full-body workout. But if you really enjoy strength training, you can easily spread it out over four or more days per week and change up the order of the muscle groups you exercise each time. Training each major muscle group twice per week is sufficient.

- What fits into your schedule now? If it is only exercising one day per week, then doing it one day per week is great. Over time, you can add more days, time, and intensity to your training once you get the hang of it all.

- It is recommended to start with 1 to 3 sets of exercises that target each major muscle group. Aim for 8 to 12 repetitions—for example, back, chest, glutes, shoulders, arms, and legs. Often, beginning with machines instead of using free weights is your best bet because they help reinforce proper alignment and form and might be safer until you feel more comfortable with the process.

■ As you begin to get more comfortable and advanced with your program and your goals become even more specific, your goals can become better defined, and you'll want to develop a specific plan tailored to help you meet those goals.

■ For example, when designing a plan to build muscle mass or improve muscle quality, there are a few things to think about and include that are unique to these plans.

   ◆ Muscular strength is a measure of how much force your muscles can produce in one effort. To improve strength, you want to do 5 to 8 repetitions at a weight that progresses up to about 80 percent of your maximal strength for 1 repetition, or 1 RM. Think higher weight and low to moderate reps for 3 sets.

   ◆ Muscular endurance ultimately leads to hypertrophy, or the increase in the muscle fiber size. For muscular endurance/hypertrophy, you would use a lower weight, roughly 65 to 85 percent of your 1 RM— for 8 to 12 repetitions and 1 to 3 sets.

   ◆ Muscular power is the amount of work performed per unit of time. This is a quick movement. Aim for a heavy load, typically more than 90 percent of your 1 RM and with only 1 to 4 repetitions.

■ To increase your muscle mass, you're going to have to put in effort when you're at the gym. If you like to lift and do aerobic exercise, that's great. And don't worry about whether you do cardio or resistance training first when you work out; it's based on personal preference.

Types of Routines

■ Assuming that you want to lift weights, you might think you should do a total-body routine or split the body segments up and work your legs one day and your upper body on a second day. But many other variations exist, such as lifting your chest and triceps on day one; then back, biceps, and shoulders on day two; and legs on day three. It can be confusing without proper guidance.

- To settle this argument, researchers recruited 20 resistance-trained young men and had them perform 2 to 3 sets of 8 to 12 reps for a total of 18 sets per session for 8 weeks. They used either a one-day-per-week split-body routine, where multiple exercises were done for 2 to 3 muscle groups per session; or a three-day-per-week total-body routine, where one exercise was performed per muscle group per session with all muscle groups trained.

- The researchers tested the upper- and lower-body strength and muscle size. After 8 weeks, there were no differences (except for greater increases in the size of the forearm flexors) in the total-body routine compared to the split-body routine.

- Select a resistance-training program that you like and can stick to— one that you think is fun and keeps you engaged. The chances of you continuing this kind of program are probably far greater than if you follow some plan that you don't think is fun.

Blood Flow Restriction

- There are other techniques that are now becoming common that are designed to help optimize muscle protein synthesis and muscle growth. If you're working with a trainer, you can discuss whether any of these would work well for you.

- One of these is called blood flow restriction, or occlusion training. Essentially, you perform low-intensity resistance training—only about 20 percent of your one-repetition maximum. You do this while also occluding blood flow with a tourniquet, or tight wrap.

- This type of training has many proposed benefits—from improved endurance during aerobic exercise, to increased muscle protein synthesis through one of the main growth-promoting signaling proteins, to the recruitment of more muscle fibers during an exercise. Some research has even shown occlusion training to increase growth hormone, which might result in beneficial physiological outcomes.

- Supporters of occlusion training say that it can produce the same responses as if you were lifting heavy weights due to the buildup up of some specific metabolites, such as adenosine monophosphate, inorganic phosphate, and lactate, as well as the depletion of phosphocreatine and a decrease in muscle pH, meaning increased acidity, or muscle "burn."

- It's not really any better than traditional training. It can be added as a supplement but shouldn't replace your normal training regimen. You might use it when you are injured and can't lift the same weight as usual. This way, you can still use light weight and get pretty good muscular adaptations.

Try This

See if you can find a great personal trainer and start lifting weights at least one time per week.

Questions to Consider

1. How will you incorporate resistance training into your exercise routine?

2. How can you modify gym-based routines for exercises at home?

Hormones and Body Composition

Your nutrition, exercise, normal physiological processes, and body composition could not occur without the help of hormones, or chemical messengers that act on specific target organs and tissues to cause cellular responses. These responses are essential to help you gain muscle and lose fat. In this lecture, you will learn about hormonal influences on body composition and consider the uncontrollable factors of sex differences and aging changes as well as the controllable factors of diet and exercise.

Insulin

- Insulin is one of the more commonly known hormones. This is because of the huge prevalence of diabetes in the United States and globally. Insulin acts on the liver, fat tissue, and muscles and is one of many hormones required for human growth and development.

- Insulin's main function is to help regulate blood sugar levels. After you eat and your blood sugar begins to rise, the beta cells of your pancreas secrete insulin, which help take glucose out of your blood and put it into cells, where it can be stored or used as energy. At the same time, insulin releases signals to your brain that you are fed, and this can act like a satiety signal, which help you feel full.

- Insulin is a storage hormone. It not only stores sugar, but it also helps you store fat. When insulin is released, it activates an enzyme called lipoprotein lipase, which not only moves fat into fat cells for storage, but also simultaneously inhibits lipolysis (fat breakdown).

- Insulin can also increase your ability to add muscle mass. This is because insulin-stimulated glucose uptake into muscle cells also enhances muscle protein synthesis by increasing the transport of amino acids into your muscles. When insulin is released, you essentially go into "storage" mode rather than "burn" mode and turn off your ability to use fat as a fuel.

■ Very high-carbohydrate meals tend to raise insulin levels the highest. Also, the glycemic index, or the relative amount that a food raises your blood glucose, can predict your insulin response. The higher the glycemic index of the carbohydrate, the more it will raise insulin.

■ This acute rise in insulin is normal and really not a problem; your body handles it, and then blood glucose and insulin will return to lower concentrations. However, if you constantly bombard your system with overloads of high-carbohydrate meals, your insulin levels will always be high. This means that you are likely spending more time in fat-storing mode than fat-burning mode.

■ If this pattern continues for long periods of time, you might become insulin resistant. This is when your cells don't respond to the insulin well, so your blood sugar is not as well controlled and your body is forced to produce more and more insulin to have the same impact on reducing your blood glucose levels.

■ It is best to avoid massive swings in insulin concentrations. Instead, aim to keep your insulin levels stable by consuming most of your carbohydrates as vegetables and whole grains. These foods tend to have lower glycemic index values—meaning that they don't raise your blood glucose very much when you eat them when compared to sweets, some breads, or juice, which have high glycemic index values.

■ Protein and fat can also influence insulin, but not to the same extent as carbohydrates. So, it might be beneficial to think about building your typical meal as protein first, good-quality fats and vegetables next, and then other low glycemic index carbohydrates.

Cortisol

- Cortisol, commonly known as the stress hormone, is often blamed for weight gain, poor health, and a slew of other headline-friendly half-truths. But the truth is that cortisol is actually very important to our overall health, helping our bodies have a healthy response to physical stressors as well as other life stressors, such as crying children, deadlines, and traffic.

- Cortisol is produced and released from the adrenal glands as part of a complex pathway known as the hypothalamic-pituitary-adrenal (HPA) axis.

- The cortisol that is released in response to normal daily patterns, or even to stress, is very useful for us metabolically. It helps us use our stored glucose, fat, and protein as energy to deal with the stresses we perceive. Additionally, cortisol can temporarily improve brain and immune function to help you overcome a fear, meet a deadline, or try new exercises.

- Cortisol also helps to decrease inflammation, which is why you might have cortisone injections into knees, wrists, and other problematic areas as you age. In fact, certain autoimmune disorders, such as rheumatoid arthritis, have been linked to a suppressed HPA axis and chronically low cortisol levels.

- Cortisol acts pretty fast. After roughly 30 minutes, cortisol will begin to degrade, and the HPA axis will stop releasing it. So, the cortisol response to an acute stress like exercise is really not all that long and is quite useful.

- Very high levels of cortisol over a long time can lead to fat storage, particularly in your visceral fat, surrounding your organs. Chronically high cortisol is also linked to psychological factors, such as depression, anxiety, and grief, and to physical factors, such as extreme levels of exercise combined with little rest and recovery.

- In these situations, not only are changes in your metabolism occurring, but your immune system might also become weak. This is why many people associate high stress or extreme exercise over a long period of time with a greater occurrence of sickness.

■ Even though exercise and other stressors can temporarily increase cortisol and cortisol in chronically elevated situations is associated with fat storage, any change in body weight or body fat is probably due to the fact that many people deal with these stresses by eating more and making bad food choices.

■ Normal levels of exercise are not likely to cause chronically high levels of cortisol. In fact, exercising for about an hour per day should help keep cortisol levels within normal ranges.

Catecholamines

■ In response to stress, exercise, or a frightening situation, many other hormones can be released. Two of these hormones are called the catecholamines, and they are also important contributors to body composition changes.

■ If you are walking through the woods and a bear walks out in front of you, your body immediately and automatically prepares you to deal with the situation. We refer to this as a "fight-or-flight response."

■ In this situation, two hormones called epinephrine and norepinephrine are secreted in high amounts into the blood. Together, these hormones are called catecholamines. They immediately provide glucose from breaking down stored glycogen and fat to your muscles so that you can either fight or run away.

■ These same responses will occur when you begin to ramp up the intensity of exercise. With intense exercise, catecholamines will be released, and you will likely notice that your heart rate and respiratory rate will increase to improve blood flow and deliver oxygen to active organs and tissues so that you can have a better fight-or-flight response.

- Catecholamines will also begin to break down stored body fat when they interact with specific receptors called adrenergic receptors, or adrenoceptors, which are receptors that respond specifically to the catecholamines.

- Because exercise and catecholamines both lead to lipolysis, or fat breakdown, exercise can be effective at burning fat as a fuel.

- One way to begin to change your body composition is to simply exercise regularly. This way, you take advantage of the catecholamine response that occurs and will lead to the breakdown of fat. But nutrition must also be considered here, along with the type and intensity of exercise being done.

- A long, slow training session would likely have the lowest catecholamine response, and if you combine this with too much food pre-exercise, during-exercise, or postexercise, then you will likely have little fat loss.

- But if you work out intensely with enough fuel to go all out but not too much that you stop lipolysis, you might have a great recipe for burning fat—in part because you have elevated your catecholamines the most with this type of workout.

- This is a trial-and-error process, though. You have to experiment with your food and your workouts to see how it makes you feel and if your body composition begins to improve over time. Then, you simply adjust accordingly to continue your path toward your optimal body composition.

- Remember, too, that if you exercise at an intense level, you might also be setting yourself up best to burn calories even after your exercise bout is finished. This "after burn" effect can last from just minutes to 24 hours, depending on your exercise intensity.

Thyroid

- The thyroid hormones also have a powerful influence on metabolism, body composition, and health. They might be the most misunderstood hormones when it comes to body composition.

- Contrary to popular belief, while thyroid problems can certainly contribute to weight gain or even weight loss, the situations where this is the primary reason for weight change are pretty rare, particularly when considering the excellent advances in medications for diagnosed thyroid problems.

- The thyroid hormones are produced by the thyroid gland, located in the front of your neck. The two hormones released from the thyroid gland are called thyroxine (T_4) and triiodothyronine (T_3). These unique messengers affect most bodily functions and influence nearly every tissue in your body throughout your entire life.

- The thyroid hormones regulate body temperature and are required for efficient metabolism, normal growth and development, and the actions of many other hormones. Without normal levels of thyroid hormones and growth hormone, for example, infants and children experience growth and developmental problems.

- Because the thyroid hormones are involved in many metabolic processes, they also play a role in maintaining and increasing your resting metabolic rate and production of body heat—a process called thermogenesis. Heat production is another process that uses energy and can influence your body composition over time.

- Many of the bodily functions that thyroid hormones influence expend energy, and we need to replenish that energy by eating. Normally, T_3 will increase energy expenditure after we eat, or "burn more calories," as our food is broken down and transported to various cells within the body. This can help regulate weight when the thyroid hormones are within a normal range.

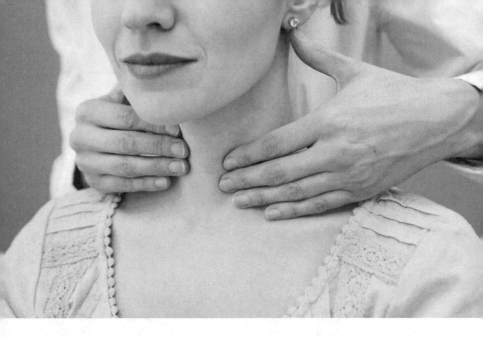

- We need to have normal T_3 levels to be healthy in a number of ways. Unfortunately, some people experience chronically low levels of T_3 and T_4, which is called hypothyroidism. In this circumstance, weight gain is likely. If the opposite occurs and T_3 and T_4 are chronically high, this is called hyperthyroidism and would likely result in weight loss.

- If you are taking medication for diagnosed hypothyroidism, then your levels are normal because of the thyroid medication that your physician has prescribed.

- Your body is capable of maintaining a healthy body composition with smart exercise and quality nutrition, as long as your thyroid levels are regulated.

Hormones, Gender, and Age

- Men naturally have more lean muscle compared to women, while women tend to have more total body fat. This is often explained by the location of body fat and the unique reproductive function needs for women. This higher level of fat and lower level of muscle in women typically means that women have metabolic rates that are about 5 to 10 percent lower than men of the same height and weight because muscle mass is more metabolically active. This might explain some of the gender discrepancies in metabolism.

■ In addition, women are 5 to 8 times more likely to develop hypothyroidism compared to men, which, if not treated, may lead to weight gain. The prevalence of hypothyroidism increases with age, too, affecting about 9 percent of men and women over the age of 60 years old. This might have implications for weight gain in later years, because a decrease in thyroid hormones slows metabolic rate if not treated with medication.

■ Additionally, decreased muscle mass and strength occurs as we get older, resulting from a gradual loss (about 5 to 10 percent per decade) of skeletal muscle after the age of 30. But these massive changes to body composition only occur if you choose not to exercise or eat properly. In fact, there is other evidence that shows excellent muscle mass quality and function in those who are lifelong exercisers and athletes.

Try This

Limit your intake of added sugars and sugar-sweetened beverages to control your insulin levels, hunger, and body composition.

Questions to Consider

1. What are the primary hormones responsible for dictating body composition?

2. What myths were put to rest in this lecture?

Novel Ways to Change Body Composition

The best method for changing body composition is by increasing the quality of both your exercise and dietary intake. But this can be complicated, leaving some people to search for outside-the-box options—such as using no-calorie sweeteners, using a stand-up desk, wearing ice-cold vests, or simply sleeping more—to help them meet their body composition goals. The rationale behind these methods is generally to either decrease the amount of food you eat or increase your total energy expenditure. This lecture is dedicated to evaluating the efficacy of some of the less-traditional approaches to altering body composition.

Artificial Sweeteners

- There are some tools and tricks that are used to decrease total energy intake to manipulate body composition. To limit calorie intake, many people choose to use low-calorie or no-calorie sweeteners.

- Originally, these artificial sweeteners were for people with diabetes because of their inability to handle large doses of real sugar, but in recent years, they have been incorporated into diets of those looking to lose weight and fat.

- While some research shows that using low-calorie sweeteners instead of full-calorie versions can improve weight loss, there have been some claims that the use of artificial sweeteners can actually increase body weight and might cause negative health effects.

- You might find success using low-calorie sweeteners in moderation to decrease energy intake and help maintain weight loss. Although more research is needed, it seems reasonable to try to choose the artificial

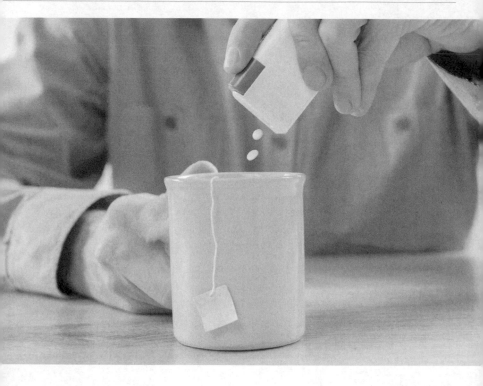

sweeteners that are as natural as you can get. For example, stevia is an herb; you can even grow it in your garden.

■ But just because they might be more natural does not mean that they are safer. It is probably best to limit added sugars or added artificial sweeteners when possible.

Detox Diets

■ Another popular dietary method that people use to try to improve body composition and weight loss is the ever-popular detox, or cleanse, diet. Detox regimens normally include pretty serious calorie restriction and focus on the consumption of fruits and vegetables only, many times in the form of juices.

- With calorie restriction, you are likely to see weight loss results, but where is this weight loss coming from? The weight loss from detox diets is most likely coming from a loss of stored glucose, also called glycogen.

- When you drastically reduce calorie intake, you will deplete glycogen stores from your body in just 24 to 48 hours, which results in even more weight loss, because glycogen is stored with water. So, you end up losing stored glucose and water weight.

- Cleanses, or detox diets, only provide short-term fixes for weight loss and do not result in long-term improvements in fat mass. They might even decrease your muscle mass, which is definitely not desirable.

- The science does not support the use of detox diets for health or body composition improvements. Until there is consistent research evidence to the contrary, with a healthy liver, you have all the detox power that you need.

Eating Out versus at Home

- Probably the easiest way to consume fewer overall calories and create a negative energy balance is to consider how much you eat out at restaurants each week.

- Research has shown that eating out at a fast-food or full-service restaurant resulted in an increase in total energy intake, saturated fat, and sodium intake. In fact, eating out results in approximately an extra 200 calories eaten per day.

- The typical American adult eats a meal or snack from a restaurant 5.8 times per week. This might cause a long-term positive energy balance, especially if you make poor choices at the restaurant and don't exercise much.

■ Even with busy schedules, making a conscious effort to prepare more meals at home might make the difference between being stuck in a plateau and reaching the goals you have set for yourself.

■ It is important to be conscious of portion sizes, regardless of whether you are eating out or cooking at home. Sometimes, you just need to practice eating until you are about 80 percent full. It can take a little while for you to realize that you've had enough to eat—sometimes as long as 15 to 20 minutes.

Sedentary Lifestyle

■ Americans spend an average of 13 hours per day with no movement. Then, if you add 8 hours of sleep, this makes it a whopping total of 21 hours per day—almost 90 percent of your day.

■ Studies have found that even if you are doing some physical activity during the day, it can't outdo the harmful effects of sitting during the other time. Sitting for an extended amount of time per day has been related to the development of cancer, diabetes, and cardiovascular disease.

■ The simple solution is to move more. Research has shown that people who take more breaks from sitting have lower waist circumferences, lower body mass indexes, and better glucose control. And the average length of the breaks was only 4.5 minutes.

■ No matter how busy you are, you can find a few minutes to get up and move. Try something simple like drinking more water so that you have to get up more to use the bathroom more often. Or instead of calling or sending an email to people in your building for a meeting, walk to their office and meet in person.

■ Even those who fidget throughout the day might see health benefits. A study from the Mayo Clinic placed sensors on people to measure their daily movement and found that people who commonly paced and fidgeted during the day—including tapping their feet, bouncing their legs, or twiddling their thumbs—were leaner than people who did not fidget as much. Those tiny movements add up over a day.

- Another option to cut down on sitting time is to use a standing desk at work, whether this is at the office or at home. You can even add a walking treadmill underneath your desk.

- Find a few minutes at lunch to walk, or make a rule to always stand up when you are on the phone. Start small and work up to standing more and more every day.

- But just standing isn't the answer, either; it is best to shift around and stand in different positions, such as having one leg up or kneeling. You can find tutorials online about the best positions to stand at your desk.

Cold Exposure

- A concept that has taken off in recent years to improve body composition is to use cold thermogenesis as a way to increase energy expenditure. There are cold vests on the market that promise you'll burn up to 500 more calories. Others say to take a cold shower, sit in an ice bath, or simply be exposed to cold environments throughout the day if you want to stay thin and lose fat.

- A 2014 study compared the metabolic effects of exercise to the metabolic effects of shivering by covering the study participants with cold water–filled blankets. The energy expenditure was higher with exercise than just being cold, but similar increases in a hormone known as irisin, which is released both during muscle contraction and during shivering, were seen in both conditions.

- Although it might increase energy expenditure slightly, there haven't been studies that show that shivering will induce weight loss or fat loss on its own. Some research exists, but the outcomes are scattered, so a more straightforward and practical examination of cold thermogenesis is needed.

Chewing

- Research has shown that when you increase the number of times you chew your food, you eat less food and also have a higher thermic effect of food. The thermic effect of food, or diet-induced thermogenesis, means that you increase energy expenditure for digestion, absorption, and storage of food.

- Although this technique might seem to have a small impact, think about how quickly you can eat your food when you're really hungry or in a rush. Odds are that you aren't paying attention and taking the time to chew your food very well.

- This method certainly isn't going to change your body overnight, but it is something to think about as you eat each meal. When you eat slowly and chew more, you might just increase the thermic effect of that meal and decrease the total number of calories you eat, too.

Sleep

- Sleep, or lack of sleep, is more crucial to weight loss and weight gain than most people realize. A 2013 Gallup poll found that 40 percent of adults are getting less than 7 hours of sleep per night, which is below the lowest recommended amount. The national average is only 6.8 hours per night.

- In addition, it is estimated that 50 to 70 million Americans have some form of sleep or wakefulness disorder, making it difficult to get a solid 8 hours per night.

- It is likely that this ambitious attitude and continuous sleep debt is hurting our health. Sleep can have an effect on metabolic control, insulin sensitivity, food cravings, muscle recovery, body composition, and hormone profile and performance. Sleep debt has also been shown to increase the risk of several chronic diseases.

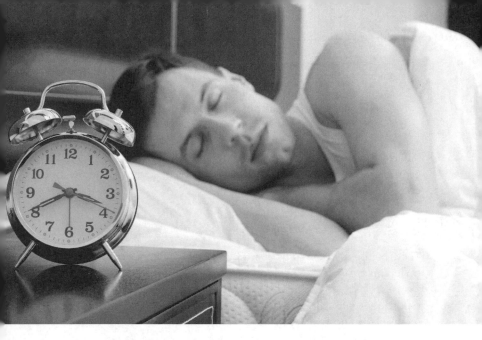

- In addition, sleep is a time for your body to heal and recover. Without proper sleep and recovery, it will be more difficult to make the body composition changes you might be looking for. Lack of sleep will cause more fatigue, making your next exercise bout more difficult. Fat loss and muscle gain will suffer.

- How can you get more sleep each night?
    - Keep a regular sleep schedule by going to bed and waking up at the same times, even on the weekends. This helps your body develop a consistent sleep-wake cycle, making it easier for you to fall asleep at night and feel more rested in the morning.
    - Manage stress and try to do something relaxing before crawling into bed each night.
    - Turn off your electronics at least 30 minutes before you try to go to sleep.
    - When you're restless, try writing down a list of things that are on your mind or wind down by reading a book.
    - Take note of what you are eating and drinking in the hours before you doze off. Because bioactive peptides naturally found in milk are

linked to more restful sleep patterns and relaxation, try drinking a small cup of milk before going to bed. It is also important to avoid certain foods and drinks before bed, such as caffeine, nicotine, or spicy foods.

- Sufficient sleep is very important, and if you don't get enough, it can seriously affect multiple systems of your body, especially body composition.

Pollutants

- There has been a new surge in attention to the influence of environmental pollutants on your body composition.

- Obesogens are chemicals in the environment that that could alter metabolism and make you have trouble losing fat. Some examples of obesogens are pesticides, pharmaceuticals, and chemicals in plastics, cans, and personal care products. One of the most common is bisphenol A, which is found in all types of plastic products.

- Obesogens are thought to disrupt your endocrine system and affect the number and size of your fat cells and other hormones associated with appetite and satiety. These alterations to the endocrine systems might result in fat gain over time.

- We don't know exactly how much exposure will make some of these compounds active in your body, so it is best to avoid exposure. When possible, try filtering water, choosing organic foods, and choosing glassware over plastic when you can.

- Exposure to pollutants is not a proven cause of metabolic issues that lead to poor body composition, but they could possibly be a contributing factor.

Try This

As much as possible, aim to get a little more sleep each night.

Questions to Consider

1. What is one nontraditional method of improving your body composition that you will try to incorporate into your routine?

2. Which of the nontraditional methods of improving body composition do you think is the most influential?

Nutrition and Exercise: Special Needs

E ven though the most common nutrition recommendations might work for many people with many different goals, there are some specific needs for certain populations. In this lecture, you will learn about plant-based eating and nutritional concerns for both young people and older people—some of the most common special dietary categories. In general, total caloric intake, protein content, micronutrient needs, and hydration status are areas to think about as you continue your quest for optimal health.

Vegetarian Eating

- A vegetarian diet is essentially a plant-based diet. There are many reasons for choosing to eat this way, and there are many ways that it's practiced in real life.

- There is a whole continuum of plant-based eating. For example, some plant-based eaters don't eat meat but do eat fish, dairy products, and eggs. Some avoid meat, fish, and eggs but will eat dairy products. Some will just avoid red meat but eat chicken and other poultry and fish. Other plant-based eaters still eat meat, just not much of it.

- The strictest form of plant-based eating is called vegan. Vegans avoid all animal products, and this includes anything that an animal might produce, such as milk, eggs, and even honey.

- Eating more plant foods is a good thing nutritionally. Typically, plants come with a good dose of fiber, vitamins, minerals, and antioxidants— molecules that help maintain your cellular health. If you are eating more plants, you likely will eat less sugar and fat. In addition, there might be fewer incidences of heart disease and cancer from eating more plants.

■ There are some very important considerations to think about when eating a plant-based diet. There is more that has to be planned and included in a plant-based diet to ensure proper intake of protein, vitamins, minerals, and more.

■ Combining sources of protein for plant-based eating is necessary to get the essential amino acids required for certain health and growth processes. The key challenge for plant-based eaters is getting the essential amino acids found in animal products into their diet.

■ Most plant sources of food have incomplete proteins; they lack one or more of the amino acids essential to maintaining and/or building your muscle tissue. But you can combine plant sources of food—such as rice and beans—to create a mixture that is complete in its protein makeup.

■ Plant-based diets might also be low in other nutrients.
  ◆ Vitamin B_{12} is only found as a "good" source in animal products. You can get B_{12} in foods like cereals that are fortified with B_{12}, but otherwise, supplementing will be needed.
  ◆ Iron is also a nutrient that needs some special attention in plant-based diets. Plant-based dieters need almost two times the amount of iron from plant sources to get the same amount of iron as meat eaters.
  ◆ Vitamin C helps you absorb plant-based iron, but calcium and tannins found in drinks like tea and coffee reduce plant-based iron absorption. Because many plant-based eaters consume a good amount of vitamin C (which is found in foods like peppers, kale, and broccoli), the absorption of iron might not be an issue. But it makes sense to combine iron intake with vitamin C and try to have calcium supplements and tea or coffee an hour or two before you eat iron-rich foods.
  ◆ Vitamin D is added to dairy foods or drinks during processing. Plant-based eaters who avoid dairy as well as meat might want to supplement with vitamin D.
  ◆ Omega-3 fats can be found in cold-water fish, but plant-based eaters can consume walnuts, seaweed, hemp, and flax. Because the

body uses the plant-based sources for omega-3 fats inefficiently, supplementation with fish oil, krill oil, or an algae-based product is needed.

◆ Calcium and zinc can be consumed in the diet, but absorption for both of these tends to be low compared to nonvegetarians. Plant-based eaters need to take in more calcium and zinc to fulfill the same requirements.

◆ If you are very physically active and trying to train for performance, consuming traditional sports supplements like creatine and beta-alanine might be something to consider.

■ On a plant-based diet, make sure that you have a combination of plant proteins to meet your goals; have a good variety of nonstarchy vegetables; include good fats; and eat starches, fruit, and starchy vegetables to complete your energy needs.

The Special Nutritional Needs of Children

■ Both children and adults need carbohydrates, fats, and proteins, but the amount needed changes as we age. The three major nutritional concerns specifically for children are sufficient calories for proper growth, development, and performance; calcium and iron intake; and hydration.

■ Active children need more calories per kilogram (or per pound) than adults do. They weigh a lot less, so their total intake is lower, but on a relative basis, children need more food per pound of body weight.

■ Dietary reference intakes (DRIs) exist for children, but they are simply baseline recommendations meant to help children live illness- and disease-free. They were not established for active children looking to perform optimally.

■ Relative to body weight, children need more protein and a higher percent of essential amino acids than adults because of their extreme rate of growth. The recommendations for boys and girls are identical, with at least 13 grams of protein per day for children ages 1 to 3, 19 grams for ages 4 to 8, and 34 grams for ages 9 to 13.

- After age 13, the recommendations differ between girls, who need at least 46 grams of protein, and boys, who need at least 52 grams of protein. This difference is mostly because boys tend to have a larger body size and larger food intake.

- A range between about 10 and 30 percent of protein in the diet is considered acceptable. Some resources recommend that children who are athletes (or at least very active) eat about 1.5 grams of protein per kilogram of body weight (or 0.7 grams of protein per pound) per day.

- Carbohydrates also come with recommendations. Children need about 130 grams per day; this provides 520 calories from carbohydrates. This might work well for your child, but you have to consider the same factors that you did for total calorie intake—especially their body size, growth rate, and activity level.

- These considerations primarily boil down to two basic recommendations: Make sure that children eat enough food, and make sure that they get enough protein to support rapid growth and development.

- Of particular concern with children is that, for the most part, they are entirely dependent on adults to purchase, prepare, and pack their food. Depending on the age of the child or adolescent, there are some pretty easy ways to have children get involved with food or cooking. Have them choose a fruit or vegetable at the store or pick a meal they want to help with.

- Another resource for children's nutrition are the DRIs of vitamins and minerals. Typically, these are lower at younger ages and progressively increase through the teenage years. Complete lists of DRIs for all age groups can be found online. Calcium and iron intake are of particular concern.

- In addition to the calorie and nutrient issues for children, their hydration needs must be considered—particularly if your child is very active. Drinking water or even diluted sports drinks is a good idea, especially during vigorous exercise and outside in warm weather.

Nutrition and Exercise with Age

- Your nutrient needs change as you age. While there is no magic drink, potion, or pill for aging, we do know that proper nutrition and exercise are vital for increasing longevity and improving quality of life as you age.

- It is not uncommon for exercise to slow down or become nonexistent as we grow older. The World Health Organization recommends at least 150 minutes of activity but says that for real benefits, it's best to exercise roughly 300 minutes per week—about 1 hour per day—for 5 days per week. This should be a mix of moderate and vigorous exercise.

- If you don't exercise now, you should start; you can add fitness, muscle, and strength at any age. Research shows that muscle quantity and quality remains excellent if physical activity is consistently part of your daily routine. In addition, it is important to eat properly not only to fuel for a healthy life, but also to help with physical activity, reduce fatigue, and maintain or build muscle mass.

- Protein intake for aging people is extremely important. According to the research on protein needs in older people, protein intake should almost be doubled compared to the recommended amount of 0.8 grams of protein per kilogram per day (or 0.36 grams per pound of body weight per day).

- This is due to the fact of an age change called anabolic resistance, where we grow resistant to the growth-promoting properties of protein. Anabolic resistance develops as early as roughly age 40.

- It is important to also include resistance training or weight lifting in your exercise plan to maintain or improve muscle mass—which is what keeps you moving and healthy. Aiming for about 30 to 40 grams of protein each time you eat might be optimal to improve muscle mass and defend against any age-related decline in muscle mass.

- You want to combine this nutrition strategy with resistance training. To fight off sarcopenia, or the age-related decline in muscle mass that affects nearly 50 percent of men and 60 percent of women aged 60 to 69 years old, you have to lift weights and eat enough calories and protein.

- Because hunger can decrease with age, it is also important to be aware of your total calorie intake.

- Two other nutrient considerations to pay attention to as you age are vitamin D and calcium. To help maintain bone mass and prevent the loss of bone, it is a good idea to eat calcium-containing foods, such as dairy products, green leafy vegetables, and fruit—or you can use a calcium

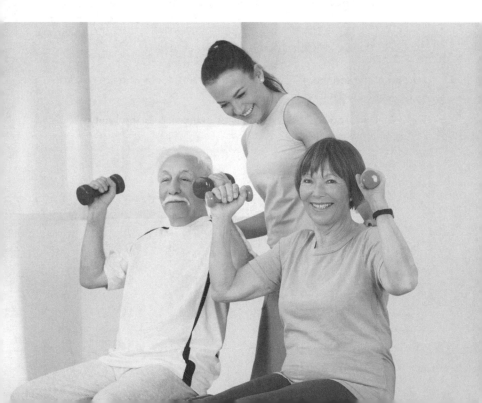

supplement. You should also make an effort to get some sun exposure or supplement with vitamin D to make sure that you are have enough to meet your needs.

■ Dehydration is also a concern in older individuals. Between the reduced ability to respond to dehydration and a reduction in thirst in older people, they can have major issues with regulating body water content. Even if you don't have the urge to drink fluids, you might need to.

Try This

Get more vegetables into your diet. Aim to eat an additional one to two servings of vegetables per day about three days per week to start.

Questions to Consider

1. What are some nutritional obstacles that people who are new to plant-based eating face?

2. What are some considerations for exercising in the heat if you are an older individual?

Set-Point Theory and the Last Five Pounds

At some point, you've probably wanted to lose "those last 5 pounds" before some upcoming event. Those last 5 pounds are often stubborn. Even with some changes that can be made to fine-tune the last 5 pounds, you'll end up fighting your physiology at some point. The set-point theory describes how and why your body is typically within just a few pounds of your "usual" body weight—the body weight that you just don't seem to budge from. In this lecture, you'll learn about ideal body weight, the set-point theory, and some common habits that make losing those last 5 pounds pretty difficult, but not impossible.

Ideal Body Weight

- Just like many topics in this field, your ideal body composition is different from that of your spouse or your best friend. Simply stop comparing and some of your stress will immediately decrease. But, of course, this is difficult to do.

- For ideal body weight, first think about what weight you were able to sustain, as an adult, where you felt the best you've ever felt. Chances are that this is more reasonable as a target then some former version of yourself with totally different life circumstances, stresses, and priorities.

- Your ideal body weight and body composition is when you feel your best, perform your best, and look your best. This ideal weight might change over time and is dependent on your goals.

- Calculating your ideal body weight is a good first step—although this will involve some trial and error.

- First, you'll need to get your body composition measured. This can be done by any of the various measurement techniques, such as a skinfold test, bioelectrical impedance analysis, or DXA scan. Your best bet is to look up exercise science labs at local universities or colleges or speak with some professional staff at your health club. Just be sure to use the same method for measuring each time.

- Once you have your body composition measured, take your weight of muscle mass and divide it by (1 – your goal body fat percent). This value is your ideal body weight at your selected percent body fat. This is your new goal weight.

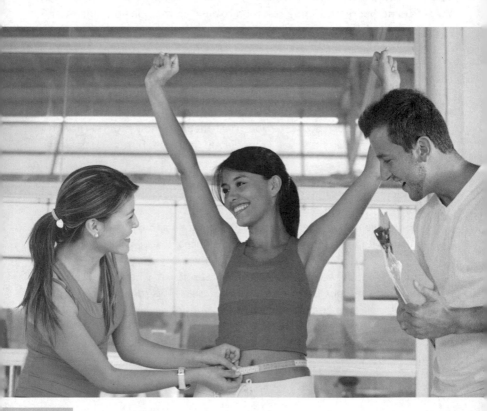

- Then, subtract your goal weight from your current weight to determine how many pounds (or kilograms) of fat you need to weigh your goal weight and have your goal body fat percent.

- This might be simple to calculate, but making it a reality is the difficult part. Despite implementing the right steps for diet and exercise, sometimes a plateau still hits you unexpectedly.

Set-Point Theory

- The concept of set point also goes by names like "lipostat" or "homeostatic control mechanism." The set-point theory states that you have a "set" weight where your body is most comfortable. By this definition, if you were to either gain or lose weight, your body would do all it could to pull you back to the original starting weight.

- For example, if you start to diet and exercise properly, it is common to lose weight rapidly at first before this rate of weight loss slows down significantly. In other words, you hit a plateau.

- While you might have great intentions and a great start to a new lifestyle, in the end, despite great efforts and initial changes, body fat and weight tend to creep back up, and there is no improved body composition or health.

- Often, if you restrict your food intake enough, it just dramatically increases your hunger levels—similar in some cases to starvation. This response is called hyperphagia, or increased hunger.

- The truth about most diets is that you eventually return to the ways you used to eat. Typically, this is because you change so many things all at once that you can't keep it up. Other times, the diets are just absurd, and you can't live a real life.

- When you do eat again after a severe diet, your fat mass comes back quickly compared to the slower development of lean muscle. You might feel hungry until your muscle mass has fully recovered. You also slow your metabolic rate, in part due to the loss of lean mass.

■ If you put together reduced energy expenditure with increased hunger, you could end up with more fat mass and body weight after dieting.

■ It seems that we are just ingrained with a body weight that our bodies work hard to defend. This is the set-point theory.

■ Essentially, you have a well-regulated internal control mechanism in the hypothalamus that tightly maintains your preset level of body fat and body weight. Your hypothalamus responds to signals from your fat cells, your gastrointestinal tract, and your pancreas to alter your metabolism, hunger, body fat levels, and weight.

■ Not only do these changes occur but you also have some hormones like ghrelin, leptin, and serotonin that control your hunger and appetite.

■ And, just as you might expect, if you lose weight, there is a good chance you'll end up hungry, and if you gain weight, you may end up losing your appetite.

■ With weight loss, your metabolic rate will decrease, so you require fewer calories than you used before you started losing weight. Eventually, the initial decrease in food you eat becomes the "normal" amount of food you require to sustain your new size.

■ Your body no longer sees that you are eating less, so there is no energy deficit. So, now, at the lower weight, you have to adjust, lowering energy intake again—that is, reducing your calories even more—to spark more weight loss.

■ The opposite is true, too: If you are trying to gain weight by eating a lot more food, you will increase your metabolic rate in an unconscious effort to bring your weight back to a set point, where it is comfortable hanging out.

- Research repeatedly shows that when overfeeding or underfeeding stops, body weight returns to its starting point. So, despite your best efforts, it is really difficult to lose fat and keep it off. But can you change your set point?

- If you can reestablish normal hormone functioning and a normal energy balance at the lower or higher target weight—by eating high-quality foods and exercising in a smart way—then your new body weight can be maintained.

- If you make the right choices to fuel yourself well with nutrient-dense, high-quality foods and live an active and healthy lifestyle, your body simply regulates your body composition for you. Maybe you just need to consistently choose foods that work with your body composition goals rather than against them.

Breaking through a Plateau

- Despite the challenge of losing fat and keeping it off, plenty of success stories exist. So, how do you reset your set point? One theory is that if you need to focus on quality foods, then you have a chance to fix the hormones that were not serving you well and begin to automatically regain control.

- Two hormones that have to do with this are insulin and leptin. Insulin is the blood glucose–lowering and fat-storing hormone, and leptin is thought of as the "stop eating" hormone. The problem with these is that people can become resistant to both of them.

- With obesity, you have a greater risk for these hormones (among others) to not work properly, and you can become resistant to their actions. This means that even with more insulin or leptin, the normal physiological responses of clearing blood glucose and stopping your hunger do not happen easily.

- Research suggests that both eating more nourishing, high-quality foods and exercising can restore normal functioning of hormones like insulin and leptin as well as improve metabolic functioning and overall health.

- There are some more ways to break through a plateau. First, consider why you are doing this. You work hard all day long; you have a lot going on in your life. Why even focus on your body composition?

- This is very personal, but you must find a real reason for why you care about feeling your best, looking your best, and performing your best. Maybe you set a small bet with a friend. This challenge keeps you accountable and motivated.

- You need to set some behavioral goals. You'll feel a sense of accomplishment by checking off the goal of working out 3 times per week instead of just focusing on the long-term goal of improving your muscle mass by 5 pounds or losing 10 pounds of fat.

- By simply focusing on the things you can control—such as what you eat, how much and how often you eat, and your workouts—you immediately have achievable goals. This is much better than going after some lofty weight loss goal or body composition change. Like most things, half the battle can just be getting started.

- None of us have time to work out, eat well, plan ahead, or make this a priority. But all of us can make time.

- Next, consider whether you are getting sloppy—with your exercise, your sleep habits, or your nutrition. Maybe you work out with a little less intensity or for a shorter duration of time than you meant to. Maybe you dropped from a solid 8 hours per night of sleep to only 5 or 6. If you follow the same plan every day, it gets pretty easy to become a bit sloppy with your usual habits.

- If breaking a plateau is important to you, you will need to rededicate yourself to exercise basics. Make sure that you are working out for the full amount of time that you promised yourself, instead of taking a bunch of breaks and counting them as exercise.

■ You need to lift weights. This is what transforms your body, adds the most muscle mass, and helps ramp up your metabolism little by little. In addition to slowing muscle loss, lifting weights might help you get past that plateau.

■ If you've hit a plateau, it's probably a good time to revisit what you do for your overall exercise plan as well and get back in the right mindset to work out.

■ Make sure that your workout is fun, entertaining, and rewarding. Recent research determined that exercise adherence and weight loss success were largely determined by your attitude toward the workout session.

■ Focus, from time to time, on the bigger reason for needing to change. Is it to be healthy enough to play with your children and grandchildren? Is it to live well rather than just to live long? These larger goals can help, although it's usually the fun of the activity and the smaller, more immediate goals that will drive your day-to-day commitment.

■ Finally, consider whether you are getting lazy with your eating habits. This could be a great time to briefly track your calories, even if you think you're eating right. Recheck your "take for granted" habits, such as your usual serving sizes. Are you putting more on your plate than usual?

■ Try to pay attention to your hunger. Pay attention to how you feel. You don't need a huge post-workout meal every day. You might consider different food choices and sizes based on how hard you actually push yourself that day.

■ Think about your activity level and your food quality; these should be your guiding principles. Once you can get your focus back for your eating habits and exercise plan, you'll probably find that you can continue to move toward your goals.

■ Make small changes, instead of massively overhauling everything at once. Don't try to start exercising every day, eat completely new foods, drink more water, eat more vegetables and fruits, and skip every happy hour all at once. Find one very easy thing to do, such as drink more water, and begin there.

Try This

Write down three things that you feel you've become a little sloppy with in your daily routine. You'll most likely identify some great places to focus on to reset your set point.

Questions to Consider

1. What nutrition and eating habits do you take for granted that can be tightened up?

2. What are the first two small changes you can make to improve your body composition?

Choosing Your Nutrition Plan

The fad diet popularity might stem from the belief that maybe there is an easy and quick way to improve body composition. It also stems from the thought that there might be one diet that is best for everyone. But this just isn't the case. Your personal preferences and physiology have a lot to do with your success of changing your body composition through diet and exercise. This lecture will highlight some interesting key points and new research for traditional diets and popular fad diets.

MyPlate

- For many years, the conventional approach to eating in the United States was to follow the Food Guide Pyramid. In fact, many countries have some pyramid design to indicate their eating recommendations. The original design had a wide base of grains, indicating that you should build a diet primarily from carbohydrates, leading up to a peak of fat and oils to use sparingly.

- In 2011, the traditional pyramid was replaced with something called MyPlate, which is an image of a plate with the food groups on it. The new plate graphic has been both praised and criticized, but it does, at least, seem to make sense to show food on a plate rather than a pyramid. It was designed to remind Americans to eat healthfully, but not necessarily to change consumer behavior.

- This guide assumes that most Americans know how to eat healthfully and that "healthfully" has a definition that is the same for everyone. In addition, just by looking at the MyPlate image, it is difficult to interpret which foods should be a priority.

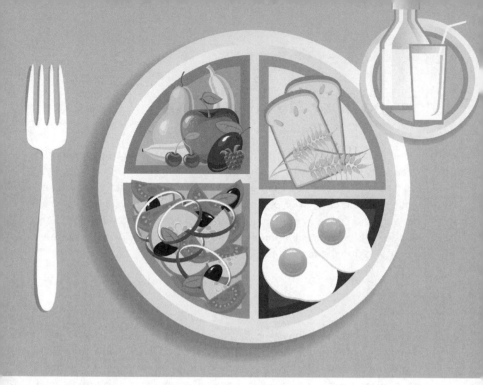

- The MyPlate recommendations encourage variety in what we eat, and they provide some visual cues for the proportion of vegetables, fruit, grains, and protein that should be on your plate. It also encourages whole grain consumption rather than simply more grain consumption.

- MyPlate recommendations, however, are very general. The MyPlate diet—traditionally thought of as a high-carbohydrate, low-fat diet—suggests that a plate 75 percent full of grains, vegetables, and fruit, which are all sources of carbohydrates, is best for everyone, regardless of how active your lifestyle is.

- For very active people, and especially people who like to work out at high intensities, a higher-carbohydrate diet has been supported in the research more times than not. This, though, is usually based on improving exercise or sports performance, but not everyone is concerned with performance. You might be much more interested in body weight or body composition.

■ The overall calorie and carbohydrate needs of someone who is physically active will be different from someone of the same size and gender who is sitting still all day at a desk.

■ In addition, constantly high blood sugar levels—which you might get following a very high-carbohydrate diet without enough exercise—are at least related to many different kinds of ailments, including type 2 diabetes.

■ Carbohydrates are not inherently a problem, but the overconsumption of them combined with a lack of physical activity tends to get people into body composition trouble.

■ The MyPlate recommendations suggest that real fruit and 100 percent fruit juice as well as real vegetables and 100 percent vegetable juices are the same. However, the ways we digest and absorb solid food compared to liquids are different in many ways, including how quickly the nutrients get into your body. In addition, many juices are loaded with added sugars that real fruit does not contain.

■ Healthy fats—such as olive oil, avocado, and fish or fish oil—are not included, even though healthy fats have a major place in our diets and have some wonderful health benefits.

■ Another drawback is that there is not really a distinction between "better" choices and "worse" choices of proteins or carbohydrates.

■ Most of the epidemiological scientific literature regarding health and weight loss in overweight individuals recommends consuming more healthy fats and reducing intake of refined carbohydrates. There are both positives and negatives with a high-carbohydrate, low-fat diet, and it is entirely dependent on how you feel, look, and perform when eating this way.

High-Fat, Low-Carb Diets

- Over much of the same time that we have been told that a higher-carb, low-fat diet is best for all of us, primarily from the MyPlate recommendations, obesity and diabetes rates have skyrocketed. So, naturally, people have been drawn to drastically different eating styles to see if they can improve their health and body composition.

- Thus, the high-fat, low-carb diet was born. This kind of eating goes by many names, such as Atkins, Paleo, and ketogenic diets. While these are different diets, some major similarities exist. Advocates of the high-fat, low-carb diets point to research that shows more fat oxidation (fat burning) with this kind of diet—and rapid weight loss.

- Eating a high-fat diet means that fat would make up about 60 to 75 percent of your total caloric intake. The assumption with high-fat diets is that if carbohydrate feeding lowers your ability to burn fat, then a high-fat diet would increase your ability to burn fat as a fuel.

- Overall, there is actually a lot of evidence to show improvements in health, body composition, and other physiological functions with a higher-fat, low-carb approach. For example, with this diet, there is higher fat oxidation during exercise, increased availability of free fatty acids, and increased activity of fat oxidation enzymes. Additionally, there is a reduction in enzymes involved with glycolysis—which is the breakdown of sugar to provide energy—along with reduced muscle glycogen and liver glycogen storage.

- If you can better control blood sugar with a high-fat, low-carb diet, this could be highly useful for controlling body fat and ultimately your overall body composition. Also, fat and protein tend to keep you feeling full for a longer period of time than carbohydrates alone.

- So, you can use a high-fat, low-carb approach to improve some health outcomes and maybe even body composition, but the problem is that this diet is often carried out incorrectly. While on a high-fat diet, people are usually just eating more fast food, fried food, and processed meats—a high fat intake, with no concern of the type of fat, along with a normal amount of carbohydrate intake. Ultimately, with a plan like this, health does not seem to improve.

- Additionally, there are some questions as to the feasibility of a high-fat, low-carb diet when you bring exercise into the equation. Some studies show no difference in exercise performance after you eat a high-fat or high-carb diet; however, these studies usually involve exercise that is done at low to moderate intensities. If you exercise at high intensities, then exercise performance might decline on a high-fat diet.

Eat Better, Not Less

There are some general guidelines for changing your body composition in a healthy, effective way.

1. Aim for minimally processed foods.
2. Try for fewer refined starches and sugars.
3. Eat protein with each meal or snack.
4. Eat more fruits and vegetables.
5. Eat more good fats, such as nuts, eggs, avocado, and fish.

The Ketogenic Diet

- Traditional high-fat, low-carb diets are 60 percent fat, 20 percent carbohydrate, and 20 percent protein. But there are two very popular diets that manipulate these percentages: the ketogenic diet and the Paleo diet.

- The ketogenic diet is a more extreme version of a typical high-fat, low-carb diet. While traditional high-fat diets allow for quite a few carbohydrates in the diet, the ketogenic diet tends to restrict carbohydrate intake to around 50 grams—2 slices of whole wheat bread—of carbohydrate per day. This diet is about 5 to 10 percent carbohydrate, 80 percent fat, and the rest protein.

- The ketogenic diet attempts to put a person into nutritional ketosis, where you burn a lot of fat. Almost all of the energy you use is from fat. When you do this, ketones are produced as natural byproducts. Your organs and cells use ketones when you are in ketosis instead of glucose. This typically would happen during periods of fasting or, as in this case, extreme carbohydrate restriction.

- The ketogenic diet is being studied for possible use as a treatment for conditions like epilepsy and even brain cancer, as well as body composition and health improvements.

- Eating like this, with so little carbohydrate, might be difficult for the first few weeks. Reports of irritability, hunger, and lethargy are common. But experts say that it becomes easier over time, and you can still exercise, perform, think, and concentrate on this kind of diet. But this is definitely not for everyone.

The Paleo Diet

- The Paleo diet is a dietary approach based on eating like we imagine our ancestors did to stay healthy, lean, and fit. The idea is that we evolved to eat certain foods but not others.

- The Paleo diet emphasizes animal products, nuts and seeds, fruits, and vegetables. Notably, strict followers of the Paleo diet do not eat grains, legumes (such as beans and peas), or dairy products. This is because the designers of the diet say that these foods did not exist 10,000 years ago, and our ancestors did not eat them. It's a sort of radical back-to-nature approach.

- Many excellent books and websites dig into the evolution of these Paleo theories, and most do not hold up to scientific scrutiny from evolutionary biologists and archaeologists (because we don't know exactly what foods our ancestors ate 10,000 years ago). Nevertheless, the Paleo diet, overall, is an approach worth considering, but likely not for the reasons that Paleo followers promote.

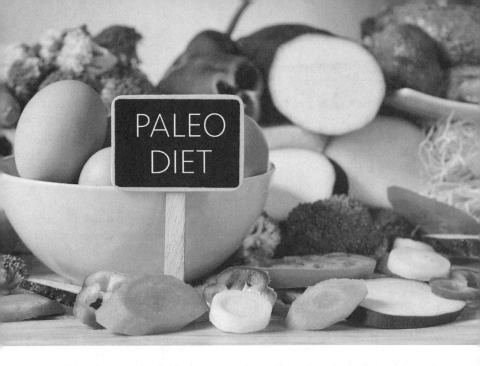

- In general, Paleo promotes good-quality foods. Research has also shown that the Paleo diet improves many markers of health and metabolism. This diet promotes quality protein intake and lots of vegetables. Whole foods are also emphasized, so this diet is superior to a typical fast-food diet.

- The exclusion of milk, legumes, and grains isn't a one-size-fits-all approach. Those with allergies or sensitivities might fair well, but for everyone else, it doesn't make much sense to eliminate all of these great foods. There are many lean, energetic, and active healthy people who choose to include milk, legumes, and dairy in their diets.

- The original Paleo diet has been revised and has changed to a much more reasonable approach that is now mainstream. Things like grass-fed dairy and some starches and wine are allowed.

Intermittent Fasting

- Intermittent fasting is simply a diet plan where you go for extended periods of time without eating. There are many types of intermittent fasting schedules. Some popular ones include alternate-day fasting, where you only eat every other day; eat, stop, eat, where you have a 24-hour fast about 1 to 2 times per week; and the 16:8 diet, where you fast for 16 hours and then have 8 hours where eating is allowed.

- Intermittent fasting is not a new concept. Most people fast for about 8 to 10 hours every night. There are religious observances, such as Ramadan, where Muslims fast from sunrise to sunset for an entire month.

- Research is now accumulating to show some benefits to following an intermittent fasting diet. Health benefits—such as improved blood lipids and blood glucose, reduced inflammation in the body, and improved appetite control—have been shown.

- Theoretically, intermittent fasting could make a difference in body composition. The problem is that there are so many different styles of fasting, so clear-cut answers are difficult to come by.

- For some people, intermittent fasting fits well into their lifestyle. If you don't like breakfast and can't be bothered to take a lunch break, it might work for you. But for others, this style of eating can promote some binge eating at night and less control over what is eaten when you finally get home, feeling starved.

- If you are exercise training while fasted, and you do this regularly, data shows elevated markers of muscle damage and overall stress. And almost all data shows a performance advantage from eating food prior to exercise and a performance decrease if you are fasted.

- The benefits reported with intermittent fasting have also been shown with exercise and a restriction-free diet. So, only choose intermittent fasting if you know it fits your lifestyle and you know you can stick to it.

Try This

Rather than a fad diet, choose a healthy eating habit that you've learned and start by fitting it into your schedule just two times per week.

Questions to Consider

1. What are the positive and negative aspects of a diet that you have tried? Was the diet successful?

2. What would be the first easy-to-change habit that you would focus on?

Motivation to Change Your Body Composition

The goal of this course has been to provide you with tools to implement change as you see fit. What you now have is a knowledge base and a tool set. Together, they offer a way to achieve more and live life as a fit and healthy person. You have the science behind the basics of nutrition and exercise and how they work to alter your body composition, improve your performance, and optimize your health. But how do you best implement these changes? This lecture discusses major motivational concepts and ideas for how to change your daily behaviors to reach your optimal body composition, health, and performance.

Successfully Changing Your Body Composition

- Changing your exercise habits alone is probably not enough to drastically change your body composition. To significantly change body composition, both smart exercise and a healthy diet are necessary.

- In addition, the type of exercise you do makes a difference. For example, research has shown that simply eating a higher-protein diet and doing both resistance training and HIIT training leads to more body fat and belly fat loss compared to eating a more traditional lower-protein diet and simply walking or jogging most days of the week.

- If your goal is to improve body composition, simplify both your diet and exercise routine, and do not change everything at once. Creating a complex meal plan and exercise schedule does you no good if you can't stick to it. It might just set you up for failure and disappointment.

- No change is too small. And the more confident you are with your goal, the more likely you are to be successful.

- Another strategy is to simply be aware and fully present when you make nutrition and exercise choices. This is more difficult than it seems.

- How many times do you try to eat a meal, finish a few emails, take a call, watch television, and talk to your spouse all at the same time? If you're too busy and distracted to pay attention to what you're eating and drinking throughout the day, it is easy to overeat or overdrink.

- Researchers have shown that distracted eating leads to eating more food at that meal and in subsequent meals. In addition, simply being mindful—or paying attention—leads to eating less later in the day.

- The type of distraction that leads to more food consumption is probably individualized. But there are many different types of mindless acts that can sabotage everything you have worked so hard for during your workouts.

- The simple act of paying attention and being physically and mentally present when you eat can make a real difference in the number of calories you consume. It's much easier to eat until you are about 80 percent full if you pay attention. There is no clear way for how to only eat until you are 80 percent full, so you will have to experiment with this.

- Research has shown that people who know about and practice being fully present when they eat—called mindful eating—take in fewer calories throughout the day and lose significantly more weight than people who do not.

- To start, slow down. Simply eating slowly might give your brain a chance to process your hunger cues and help you figure out when to stop eating. It takes a little time to feel full. If you don't give yourself that time and just keep shoveling your food in, it's pretty easy to get a few hundred extra calories down in just a few minutes.

■ Also, try to eliminate distractions. Just like when you drive, if you can stop all the distractions—such as television, tablets, cell phones, and any number of gadgets—when you eat, you'll have a better chance of making it to your destination.

■ You can also practice being fully present and engaged during your workouts. If you're outside, try to look around a bit (safely, of course) and notice the landscape and trees and smell the fresh air. If you always jog or run with music, then from time to time, try unplugging and listening to your breathing and heartbeat as you exercise.

■ Think about what muscles are working and what these exercises are doing for you. Think about how much stronger you are becoming both physically and mentally from each successful workout.

■ Some people call this the mind-body connection. You think about your progress, the blood flowing through your body and nourishing your cells, and the fuel you ate to power your workout and make you strong and energetic.

■ This ability to focus and connect with your workout could be the one thing that turns the corner for you and makes you truly love being physically active.

■ Also, find activities that you enjoy doing. They might be traditional things, such as walking, running, or swimming, or other options, such as yoga, hiking, group exercise, or sports. There are endless options for getting in your recommended amount of exercise, and it doesn't have to be something you dread.

■ To improve health, you need to exercise. Doing a wide variety of exercises, including resistance training and high-intensity intervals, can be pretty simple to include and can also be fun, especially if you are in the right mindset for change.

- Adherence to your diet and exercise plans are going to make or break your efforts. No matter the diet or exercise regimen, a participant's adherence to the program is most strongly associated with their weight loss. Simply making changes that you can stick to is the key to success with body composition change.

Grocery Shopping Tips

- One way to improve adherence is to understand how to set up your home for success, and it starts with knowing some grocery shopping tips. This is one of the most fundamental concepts that sets the stage for making successful dietary changes. If your grocery shopping is organized, it makes it so much easier for you to make better and healthier choices at home.

- Make a list before you go to the store. You arrive prepared, and you save time. Just get what you need. If it isn't on the list, don't buy it. This doesn't mean to exclude any items that you consider treats—but only buy small amounts, because if it's in your house, you'll probably eat it.

- Making a list also helps you think about your meals for the week, rather than just one meal or one day's meals. You have a broader perspective on your dietary choices. Making a list helps you prepare for meals in advance so that you're more likely to have a go-to option that fuels you right.

- If you don't use a list, especially if you are new to eating well, you are more likely to buy the food you've always bought, and that might be the problem. Use a list to remind you of the healthier choices you want to start making.

- Don't get confused by labels like "natural," "gluten-free," and "low-fat." The food industry bombards you with thousands of options, which leads to confusion and often poor choices. The health halo effect occurs when you see a label on the front of a package that says "good source of vitamin C" and believe that it is automatically better for you or lower in calories.

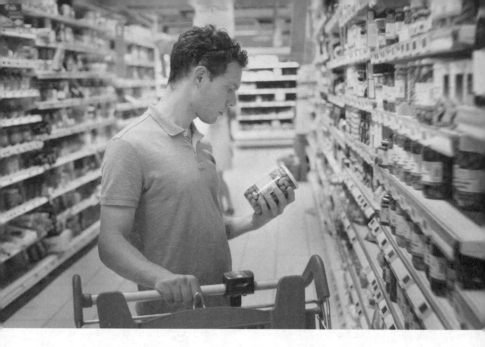

- These claims can actually mean very little, but we often believe that they are better for us. Your best bet is to investigate the product for yourself by looking at the Nutrition Facts label that can be found on each item. Or, better yet, aim for minimally processed foods with as few ingredients as possible.

- It isn't practical to think that you can avoid processed foods altogether. Almost everything we buy to eat is processed in some way. But aim for products that require the least amount of processing to get onto your plate.

- When you get home, you might even immediately wash and cut fruits and vegetables and store them in a visible place or keep a bowl of fruit out on the counter for an easy grab-and-go option. Keep things like nuts, seeds, and vegetables accessible for snacks.

- Simple changes to your grocery habits and kitchen setup will enable you to make better choices and help you meet your goals. Several facets of your lifestyle play a role in your ability to successfully make behavior changes, so take note of these and slowly address them over time.

What Progress Looks Like

- As you implement one change at a time, you might wonder what sort of results you can anticipate. Patience is key. If it took 20 years to put on, give it more than 20 days to come off.

- Losing massive amounts of weight quickly might not be the best approach. If you lose 5 pounds (2.3 kilograms) in a week, it is most likely due to changes in water weight or even from muscle loss with extreme calorie restriction. Neither of these will result in the positive body composition changes you are looking for.

- Some research supports the idea that slower weight loss might be best for actual and permanent changes in body composition, particularly with your muscle mass.

- What kind of changes in numbers should you see if you make a solid effort to improve your body composition? It's difficult to say because it is so individualized, but some experts suggest that average fat loss changes are around 0.5 percent body fat loss every 4 weeks and average muscle gain is around 1 pound (0.45 kilograms) of lean mass every 4 weeks (if those are your specific goals).

- Before focusing on numbers and goals, you should consider how these changes make you feel. Is this working for your lifestyle? And then listen to your body. But if you aren't making any progress, then it is important to reevaluate and make a change that you can stick to, and begin the process again.

- Being aware of what your progress should look like and being prepared to encounter barriers and relapses are both very important to your overall success.

Try This

Write down your shopping list and take it with you to the store to stock your house with foods that support your goals.

Questions to Consider

1. What is one behavior change that you will make to overcome a barrier?

2. What is one goal that you will set yourself to achieve?

Bibliography

Websites/Online Articles

American College of Sports Medicine. "Protein Intake for Optimal Muscle Maintenance." http://www.acsm.org/docs/default-source/brochures/protein-intake-for-optimal-muscle-maintenance.pdf. [Lecture 9]

American Diabetes Association. Glycemic Index and Diabetes. http://www.diabetes.org/food-and-fitness/food/what-can-i-eat/understanding-carbohydrates/glycemic-index-and-diabetes.html. [Lecture 6]

American Heart Association. Monounsaturated Fats. http://www.heart.org/HEARTORG/GettingHealthy/NutritionCenter/HealthyEating/Monounsaturated-Fats_UCM_301460_Article.jsp#. [Lecture 7]

Ammeson, Jane. "Sleep-Friendly Foods for a Good Night's Rest." The Times. http://www.nwitimes.com/niche/get-healthy/healthy-living/sleep-friendly-foods-for-a-good-night-s-rest/article_53cee181-89d6-529c-bcc4-f63a80ad8582.html. [Lecture 20]

Andrews, Ryan. "Body Type Eating: Find Out Whether It's Right for You." Precision Nutrition (blog). http://www.precisionnutrition.com/all-about-body-type-eating. [Lecture 2]

———. "Phytates and Phytic Acid: Here's What You Need to Know." Precision Nutrition (blog). http://www.precisionnutrition.com/all-about-phytates-phytic-acid. [Lecture 10]

Anello, Robert, Joshua D'Alessandro, and Palmer Johnson. "Dietary Contaminants and Hormonal Disturbances: Is There a Link?" Mike Ormsbee (blog). http://mikeormsbee.com/dietary-contaminants-and-hormonal-disturbances-is-there-a-link/. [Lecture 20]

Antonio, Jose. "An Ode to Nutrient Timing." *International Society of Sports Nutrition.* http://www.theissnscoop.com/an-ode-to-nutrient-timing/. [Lecture 12]

Badalaty, Gina. "Obesogens: The Hidden Chemicals That Can Make Your Family Fat." *Mamavation* (blog). http://www.mamavation.com/2015/02/obesogens-hidden-chemicals-can-make-family-fat.html. [Lecture 20]

Berardi, John. "10 Lessons for Your Leanest Summer." *Precision Nutrition* (blog). http://www.precisionnutrition.com/10-lessons-for-2012. [Lecture 22]

———. "Better Version of 'My Plate': Precision Nutrition's Eating Guidelines for Clients." *Precision Nutrition* (blog). http://www.precisionnutrition.com/pn-my-plate. [Lecture 23]

Beyond Vegetarianism. "Comparison of Vitamin Levels in Raw vs. Cooked Foods." http://www.beyondveg.com/tu-j-l/raw-cooked/raw-cooked-2f.shtml. [Lecture 10]

Boston, G. "Why It's So Hard to Lose Those Last 5 Pounds." http://www.washingtonpost.com/lifestyle/wellness/why-its-so-hard-to-lose-those-last-5-pounds/2014/05/20/c15b69f2-dae4-11e3-b745-87d39690c5c0_story.html. [Lecture 22]

Brightcove. "Weight Loss: Where Do Our Calories Go?" Video. http://link.brightcove.com/services/player/bcpid1954212222001?bckey=AQ~~,AAAB xqEDkXE~,hmZyzKR72h2-K9-NOFee3eDD2vff8t15&bctid=3571710062001. [Lecture 3]

Bushak, Lecia. "Obese People Have an Extremely Low Chance of Recovering Normal Body Weight: Study." *Medical Daily.* http://www.medicaldaily.com/obese-people-have-extremely-low-chance-recovering-normal-body-weight-study-343534. [Lecture 22]

Carnell, Susan. "Do You Eat Out of Boredom?" *Psychology Today.* https://www.psychologytoday.com/blog/bad-appetite/201112/do-you-eat-out-boredom. [Lecture 21]

Caroll, Aaron E. "To Lose Weight, Eating Less Is Far More Important Than Exercising More." *The New York Times.* http://www.nytimes.com/2015/06/16/upshot/to-lose-weight-eating-less-is-far-more-important-than-exercising-more.html?_r=1&abt=0002&abg=1. [Lecture 22]

Center for Science in the Public Interest. "Artificial Trans Fat: On the Way Out!" http://www.cspinet.org/transfat/. [Lecture 11]

Centers for Disease Control and Prevention. "Insufficient Sleep Is a Public Health Problem." http://www.cdc.gov/features/dssleep/. [Lecture 20]

———. *Nutrition.* www.cdc.gov/nutrition. [Lecture 7]

Cespedes, Andrea. "Calories Burned Standing vs. Sitting." *LIVESTRONG. COM.* http://www.livestrong.com/article/73916-calories-burned-standing-vs.-sitting/. [Lecture 16]

Dunham, Will. "Weight of the World: 2.1 Billion People Obese or Overweight." *Reuters.* http://www.reuters.com/article/2014/05/28/us-health-obesity-idUSKBN0E82HX20140528. [Lecture 6]

EatingWell (blog). "How to Set Up Your Kitchen for Weight-Loss Success." http://www.eatingwell.com/nutrition_health/weight_loss_diet_plans/how_to_set_up_your_kitchen_for_weight_loss_success?page=2. [Lecture 24]

Ericson, John. "75% of Americans May Suffer from Chronic Dehydration, According to Doctors." http://www.medicaldaily.com/75-americans-may-suffer-chronic-dehydration-according-doctors-247393. [Lecture 10]

Esco, Michael R. "Resistance Training for Health and Fitness." *American college of Sports Medicine.* http://www.acsm.org/docs/brochures/resistance-training.pdf. [Lecture 18]

Fisher, Adjua. "5 Totally Weird Science-Backed Ways to Burn Calories Today (without Exercising)." *Be Well Philly.* http://www.phillymag.com/be-well-philly/2015/03/04/5-science-backed-ways-burn-calories-today-without-exercising/. [Lecture 20]

Ghose, Tia. "Cold-Weather Benefit: Shivering May Count as Exercise." *Live Science.* http://www.livescience.com/43085-shivering-triggers-exercise-response.html. [Lecture 20]

Gorksi, Chris. "What Should Athletes and the Rest of Us Eat at Night?" *Mike Ormsbee* (blog). http://mikeormsbee.com/what-should-athletes-and-the-rest-of-us-eat-at-night/. [Lecture 13]

Greenfield, Ben. "How Much Should You Drink during Exercise?" http://www.quickanddirtytips.com/health-fitness/exercise/how-much-should-you-drink-during-exercise?page=1. [Lecture 10]

Grover, Jenni. "Mindful Eating: 5 Easy Tips to Get Started." *Huffpost Healthy Living.* http://www.huffingtonpost.com/2013/11/12/mindful-eating-tips_n_3941528.html. [Lecture 24]

Harvard Health Publications. *Glycemic Index and Glycemic Load for 100+ Foods.* http://www.health.harvard.edu/newsweek/Glycemic_index_and_glycemic_load_for_100_foods.htm. [Lecture 6]

Helland, L. "35 Lessons from Precision Nutrition's Most Successful Clients." http://www.precisionnutrition.com/35-ways-to-transform-your-body?utm_source=35WaysToTransformBody&utm_medium=Email&utm_campaign=35WaysToTransformBodyEmail. [Lecture 22]

Iowa State University Extension and Outreach. *Fat.* http://www.extension.iastate.edu/humansciences/fat. [Lecture 7]

Ji, Sayer. "Splenda (Sucralose) Found to Have Diabetes-Promoting Effects." *Epoch Times.* http://www.theepochtimes.com/n3/1162919-splenda-sucralose-found-to-have-diabetes-promoting-effects/. [Lecture 20]

Jones, Jeffrey M. "In U.S., 40% Get Less Than Recommended Amount of Sleep." *Gallup.* http://www.gallup.com/poll/166553/less-recommended-amount-sleep.aspx. [Lecture 20]

Keller, Tracy. "The Psychology behind a Grocery Store's Layout." *Notre Dame College Online.* http://online.notredamecollege.edu/psychology/the-psychology-behind-a-grocery-store%E2%80%99s-layout/. [Lecture 24]

Kirkpatrick, Kristin. "5 Strategies to Help You Stop Emotional Eating." *Health Essentials.* http://health.clevelandclinic.org/2015/05/5-strategies-to-help-you-stop-emotional-eating/. [Lecture 24]

Kotulak, R. "Vitamin a Day Just What the Doctor Orders." *Chicago Tribune.* http://articles.chicagotribune.com/2002-06-19/news/0206190305_1_vitamins-rdas-pellagra. [Lecture 10]

Kotz, Deborah. "Are No-Calorie Sweeteners Safe to Eat?" *The Boston Globe.* https://www.bostonglobe.com/lifestyle/health-wellness/2014/01/27/are-calorie-sweeteners-safe/B56kqUuKVJwcEfcWx2PmhO/story.html. [Lecture 20]

Kravitz, Len, and Vivian H. Heyward. "Getting a Grip on Body Composition." http://www.unm.edu/~lkravitz/Article%20folder/underbodycomp.html. [Lecture 2]

Kuzma, Cindy. "The New Math of Calorie Counting." *Men's Health.* http://www.menshealth.com/weight-loss/counting-calories-weight-loss?cm_mmc=DailyDoseNL-_-1755306-_-06302014-_-TheNewMathofCalorieCounting-hed. [Lecture 22]

MacMillan, Amanda. "11 Ways to Stop Overeating after Your Workout." *Time.* http://time.com/3341969/overeating-after-your-workout/. [Lecture 22]

Marie, Joanne. "A List of Leucine-Rich Foods." *LIVESTRONG.COM.* http://www.livestrong.com/article/346375-a-list-of-leucine-rich-foods/ nutritiondata.com. [Lecture 8]

Matilda, Benita. "Increased Chewing Benefits Weight Management." *Science World Report.* http://www.scienceworldreport.com/articles/14587/20140509/increased-chewing-one-of-the-benefiting-weight-management-strategy.htm. [Lecture 20]

May, Kyle P. "What Are METs on a Treadmill?" *LIVESTRONG.COM.* http://www.livestrong.com/article/49231-mets-treadmill/. [Lecture 16]

Mayo Clinic. "Resveratrol in Grapes, Supplements and Other Foods." http://www.mayoclinic.org/diseases-conditions/heart-disease/in-depth/red-wine/art-20048281?pg=2. [Lecture 10]

———. "Sleep Tips: 7 Steps to Better Sleep." http://www.mayoclinic.org/healthy-lifestyle/adult-health/in-depth/sleep/art-20048379?pg=2. [Lecture 20]

Mendez, Elizabeth. "Americans Continue to Adjust Their Ideal Weight Upward." *Gallup.* http://www.gallup.com/poll/158921/americans-continue-adjust-ideal-weight-upward.aspx?utm_source=google&utm_medium=rss&utm_campaign=syndication. [Lecture 2]

Migala, Jessica. "10 Types of Hunger and How to Control Them." *Fox News.* http://www.foxnews.com/health/2014/08/30/10-types-hunger-and-how-to-control-them/. [Lecture 22]

Mosley, Michael. "Calorie Burner: How Much Better Is Standing Up Than Sitting?" *BBC News.* http://www.bbc.com/news/magazine-24532996. [Lecture 16]

Mozaffarian, D. "Dietary Priorities for Preventing Obesity: Are All Calories Created Equal?" https://www.youtube.com/watch?v=GHTsJR0fuIs&feature=youtu.be. [Lecture 23]

MyFoodDiary.com. *Exercise and Avoiding Dehydration.* http://www.myfooddiary.com/resources/ask_the_expert/exercise_avoiding_dehydration.asp. [Lecture 10]

National Heart, Lung, and Blood Institute. *Calculate Your Body Mass Index.* http://www.nhlbi.nih.gov/health/educational/lose_wt/BMI/bmicalc.htm. [Lecture 2]

————. *Portion Distortion: Do You Know How Food Portions Have Changed in 20 Years?* https://www.nhlbi.nih.gov/health/educational/wecan/eat-right/portion-distortion.htm. [Lecture 1]

National Institutes of Health. *Vitamin A.* http://ods.od.nih.gov/factsheets/VitaminA-HealthProfessional/. [Lecture 10]

————. *Vitamin and Mineral Supplement Fact Sheets.* www.cc.nih.gov/ccc/supplements. [Lecture 10]

Nestle, Marion. "FDA's New Food Label: Much Improved!" *Food Politics* (blog). http://www.foodpolitics.com/2014/02/fdasnew-food-label-much-improved/. [Lecture 11]

Newman, Hannah. "Why Not Even Exercise Will Undo the Harm of Sitting All Day—And What You Can Do About It." *Quartz.* http://qz.com/223160/why-not-even-exercise-will-undo-the-harm-of-sitting-all-day-and-what-you-can-do-about-it/. [Lecture 20]

Nierenberg, Cari. "Why Diets Fail: Your Feelings May Dictate Food Choices." *Live Science.* http://www.livescience.com/50803-diets-fail-feelings-food-choices.html. [Lecture 24]

Nutrition.gov. "Questions to Ask before Taking Vitamin and Mineral Supplements." http://www.nutrition.gov/dietary-supplements/questions-ask-taking-vitamin-and-mineral-supplements. [Lecture 10]

Ormsbee, Mike. "Healthy Shopping Tips at the SuperMarket.flv." Video. https://www.youtube.com/watch?v=XA0QCN3YQDI. [Lecture 24]

Orwell, Sol. "Detoxes: An Undefined Scam." *Examine* (blog). http://examine.com/blog/detoxes-an-undefined-scam/?utm_source=Examine.

com+Insiders&utm_campaign=f11d8e46c5-email_Detox1_21_2015&utm_medium=email&utm_term=0_e4d662cb1b-f11d8e46c5-69935085&goal=0_e4d662cb1b-f11d8e46c5-69935085&mc_cid=f11d8e46c5&mc_eid=1ba8bb7558. [Lecture 20]

Pennington Biomedical Research Center. *Single Subject Weight Change Predictor.* http://www.pbrc.edu/research-and-faculty/calculators/sswcp/.

Persistence Market Research. "Sports Nutrition Market Will Reach $37.7 Billion in 2019, Globally." *Globe Newswire.* http://globenewswire.com/news-release/2014/09/23/667761/10099668/en/Sports-Nutrition-Market-Will-Reach-37-7-Billion-in-2019-Globally-Persistence-Market-Research.html. [Lecture 14]

PR Newswire. "New Survey: To Sit or Stand? Almost 70% of Full Time American Workers Hate Sitting, but They do it All Day Every Day." http://www.prnewswire.com/news-releases/new-survey-to-sit-or-stand-almost-70-of-full-time-american-workers-hate-sitting-but-they-do-it-all-day-every-day-215804771.html. [Lecture 20]

Precision Nutrition. "Kitchen Makeover Questionnaire." http://www.precisionnutrition.com/wordpress/wp-content/uploads/2014/11/precision-nutrition-fitpro-starter-kit-assess.pdf. [Lecture 24]

Rosenbrock, Katie. "Give Up These 5 Things to Get Rid of Your Gut for Good." *The Active Times.* http://www.theactivetimes.com/give-these-5-things-get-rid-your-gut-good. [Lecture 22]

Science Clarified. *Lympatic System.* http://www.scienceclarified.com/Io-Ma/Lymphatic-System.html#ixzz3U0bzXGGg. [Lecture 3]

SELFNutritionData. *Nutrition Facts.* http://nutritiondata.self.com/facts/vegetables-and-vegetable-products/2626/2. [Lecture 11]

Smith, Michael A. "Can Lack of Sleep Lead to Carb Cravings?" *Life Extension* (blog). http://blog.lifeextension.com/2011/08/can-lack-of-sleep-lead-to-carb-cravings.html?utm_campaign=normal&utm_source=twitter&utm_medium=social&m=1. [Lecture 20]

St. Pierre, Brian. "Is Nutrient Timing Dead? And Does 'When' You Eat Really Matter?" *Precision Nutrition* (blog). http://www.precisionnutrition.com/nutrient-timing. [Lecture 12]

———. "The Paleo Problem: Examining the Pros and Cons of the Paleo Diet." *Precision Nutrition* (blog). http://www.precisionnutrition.com/paleo-diet. Site visit 8/12/2015. [Lecture 23]

Stone Hearth News. "Eating Out, No Matter Where, Adds 200 Calories a Day." http://www.stonehearthnewsletters.com/eating-matter-adds-200-calories-day/junk-food/#sthash.WbGzT32z. [Lecture 20]

———. "Green, Black, and Oolong Tea Polyphenols May Reduce Visceral Fat, Inflammation." http://www.stonehearthnewsletters.com/green-black-oolong-tea-polyphenols-may-reduce-visceral-fat-inflammation/inflammation/. [Lecture 20]

———. "Not Splendid News for Splenda, Sukrana, SucraPlus, Candys, Cukren and Nevella." http://www.stonehearthnewsletters.com/splendid-news-splenda-sukrana-sucraplus-candys-cukren-nevella/nutrition-food-artificial-sweeteners/. [Lecture 20]

Stromberg, Joseph. "Five Health Benefits of Standing Desks." *Smithsonian.* http://www.smithsonianmag.com/science-nature/five-health-benefits-standing-desks-180950259/?no-ist. [Lecture 16]

Sucralose. "New Research Analyzing 35 Years of Data Confirms Positive Effects of Low-Calorie Sweeteners in Weight Loss." http://sucralose.org/new-research-analyzing-35-years-of-data-confirms-positive-effects-of-low-calorie-sweeteners-in-weight-loss/. [Lecture 20]

SuppVersity (blog). "Can You Become Fat in Only 3 Days? Even with 1,500 Extra Calories, You Can't. All But One Subject Actually Lost Some Body Fat during 3-Day Gluttony on > 50% CHO Diets!" http://suppversity.blogspot. com/2014/09/can-you-get-fat-in-three-days-study.html. [Lecture 22]

———. "Food Is Medicine: Each 10g Fiber Reduce Mortality Risk by up to 34%! Phenols Battle Alzheimer's & Breast Cancer & Two Dozen Dietary GLUT4 Boosters Prevent Diabetes." http://suppversity.blogspot.de/2015/01/food-is-medicine-each-10g-fiber-reduce.html. [Lecture 10]

———. "Prevalent Nutrient Deficiencies in the US: More Than 40% Are Vitamin A, C, D & E, Calcium or Magnesium Deficient and > 90% Don't Get Enough Choline, Fiber & Potassium." http://suppversity.blogspot. com/2015/01/prevalent-nutritient-deficiencies-in-us.html?m=1. [Lecture 10]

Tartar, Jaime. "In Defense of Cortisol." *International Society of Sports*. http:// www.theissnscoop.com/in-defense-of-cortisol/. [Lecture 19]

The University of New Mexico Health Sciences Center. "Stairway to Health." http://hsc.unm.edu/wellness/physical/stairs.html. [Lecture 16]

U.S. Food and Drug Administration. *Dietary Supplement Labeling Guide: Chapter IV. Nutrition Labeling.* http://www.fda.gov/Food/ GuidanceRegulation/GuidanceDocumentsRegulatoryInformation/ DietarySupplements/ucm070597.htm#4-3. [Lecture 14]

———. "Proposed Label/What's Different?" http://www.fda.gov/downloads/ Food/GuidanceRegulation/GuidanceDocumentsRegulatoryInformation/ LabelingNutrition/UCM387451.pdf. [Lecture 11, Lecture 15]

———. *Proposed Changes to the Nutrition Facts Label.* http://www.fda. gov/Food/GuidanceRegulation/GuidanceDocumentsRegulatoryInformation/ LabelingNutrition/ucm385663.htm. [Lecture 11]

Walton, Alice G. "How Much Sugar Are Americans Eating?" *Forbes*. http:// www.forbes.com/sites/alicegwalton/2012/08/30/how-much-sugar-are-americans-eating-infographic/. [Lecture 20]

Wood, Sheryl. "Timing of Weight Loss Efforts Matters." *Daily Rx News.* http://www.dailyrx.com/exercise-first-then-diet-prevented-muscle-loss-people-metabolic-syndrome. [Lecture 22]

Zelman, Kathleen M. "Fiber: How Much Do You Need?" *Web MD.* http://www.webmd.com/food-recipes/features/fiber-how-much-do-you-need. [Lecture 6]

Zuckerbrot, Tanya. "5 Ways to Bust a Diet Plateau." *Fox News.* http://www.foxnews.com/health/2014/05/13/5-ways-to-bust-diet-plateau/. [Lecture 22]

Printed Works/Books

Antonio, J., D. Kalman, J. R. Stout, M. Greenwood, D. S. Willoughby, and G. G. Haff. *Essentials of Sports Nutrition and Supplements.* New York: Humana Press, 2008. This is the textbook for the undergraduate course in sports nutrition and sports supplements. [Lecture 5]

Bailor, Jonathan. *The Calorie Myth.* New York: HarperCollins Publishers, 2014. According to this author, by focusing on food and exercise quality rather than calorie quantity, you can burn fat and boost health more easily and enjoyably than you ever thought possible. [Lecture 11, Lecture 22]

Berardi, J., and R. Andrews. *The Essentials of Sport and Exercise Nutrition Certification Manual.* 2nd ed. Toronto, ON: Precision Nutrition, 2010. This is a companion workbook that is meant to accompany a nutritional certification program called Precision Nutrition. [Lecture 1, Lecture 6, Lecture 7, Lecture 8, Lecture 15]

Greenfield, Ben. *Beyond Training: Mastering Endurance, Health & Life.* Riverside, NJ: Victory Belt Publishing, 2014. Offers advice regarding health and lifestyle. [Lecture 5, Lecture 23]

Gropper, S. S., J. L. Smith, and J. L. Groff. *Advanced Nutrition and Human Metabolism.* Edited by P. Adams, A. Lustig, and E. Feldman. Belmont, CA:

Wadsworth/Cengage Learning, 2009. Covers the biochemistry of vitamins, minerals, and energy nutrients. [Lecture 3, Lecture 4, Lecture 19]

Hadley, M. E., and J. E. Levine. *Endocrinology.* 6th ed. Upper Saddle River, NJ: Pearson Prentice Hall, 2007. Offers applications and in-depth coverage of vertebrate hormones. [Lecture 19]

Lieberman, Michael, and Allan D. Marks. *Mark's Basic Medical Biochemistry: A Clinical Approach.* Edited by Susan Rhymer. Baltimore, MD: Lippincott Williams & Wilkins, 2013. Offers a patient-oriented approach that links biochemistry to physiology and pathophysiology.

Mahan, L. K., S. Escott-Stump, and J. L. Raymond. *Krause's Food and the Nutrition Care Process.* St. Louis, MO: Elsevier Saunders, 2012. Provides up-to-date information about nutrition. [Lecture 19]

McArdle, William D., Frank I. Katch, and Victor L. Katch. *Sports and Exercise Nutrition.* 4th ed. Philadelphia, PA: Lippincott Williams & Wilkins, 2012. Offers nutrition and exercise concepts and their practical applications. [Lecture 1, Lecture 5]

McClusky, Mark. *Faster, Higher, Stronger.* New York: Hudson Street Press, 2014. The author explains how today's top athletes are turning to advanced technology and savvy science to improve their performance. [Lecture 23]

Moore, J., and E. Westman. *Keto Clarity: Your Definitive Guide to the Benefits of a Low-Carb, High-Fat Diet.* Riverside, NJ: Victory Belt Publishing, 2014. Explains the powerful therapeutic effects of a ketogenic diet. [Lecture 23]

Straub, R. O. *Health Psychology: A Biopsychosocial Approach.* 3rd ed. New York: Worth Publishers, 2012. With an emphasis on positive health, the new edition examines information from biological, psychological, and social aspects of health. [Lecture 19]

Volek, J., and S. Phinney. *The Art and Science of Low Carbohydrate Performance.* Miami, FL: Beyond Obesity, 2012. Presents more than 130 recipes. [Lecture 22]

Journal Articles

Acheson, K. J., et al. "Protein Choices Targeting Thermogenesis and Metabolism." *American Journal of Clinical Nutrition* 93, no. 3 (2011): 525–534. The objective of this study was to determine the differential effects of three proteins on energy metabolism, satiety, and glucose control. [Lecture 1]

Agarwal, S., et al. "Comparison of Prevalence of Inadequate Nutrient Intake Based on Body Weight Status of Adults in the United States: An Analysis of NHANES 2001–2008." *Journal of the American College of Nutrition* 34, no. 2 (2015): 126–134. The objective of this study was to compare micronutrient intake status of overweight and obese adults with normal-weight adults. [Lecture 10]

Ahmed, T., and N. Haboubi. "Assessment and Management of Nutrition in Older People and Its Importance to Health." *Journal of Clinical Interventions in Aging* 5 (2010): 207–216. Nutrition is an important element of health in the older population and affects the aging process. [Lecture 3]

Alfenas, Rde C., J. Bressan, and A. C. Paiva. "Effects of Protein Quality on Appetite and Energy Metabolism in Normal Weight Subjects." *Arquivos Brasileiros de Endocrinologia & Metabologia* 54, no. 1 (2010): 45–51. The goal of this study was to compare the effects of consumption of different protein sources on food intake and energy expenditure in normal-weight subjects. [Lecture 1]

American College of Sports Medicine, American Dietetic Association, and Dieticians of Canada. "Joint Position Statement: Nutrition and Athletic Performance. American College of Sports Medicine, American Dietetic Association, and Dietitians of Canada." *Medicine & Science in Sports & Exercise* 32, no. 12 (2000): 2130–2145. These three organizations have taken the position that physical activity, athletic performance, and recovery from exercise are enhanced by optimal nutrition. [Lecture 12]

Apolzan, J. W., et al. "Inadequate Dietary Protein Increases Hunger and Desire to Eat in Younger and Older Men." *Journal of Nutrition* 137, no. 6 (2007): 1478–1482. This study was designed to examine the appetitive responses to habitual protein intakes that span the range of adequacy in younger and older men. [Lecture 1]

Aragon, Alan A., and Brad Jon Schoenfeld. "Nutrient Timing Revisited: Is There a Post-Exercise Anabolic Window?" *Journal of International Society of Sports Nutrition* 10, no. 5 (2013): 1–11. The purpose of this paper is to review the existing literature on the effects of nutrient timing with respect to postexercise muscular adaptations and to draw relevant conclusions that allow practical nutritional recommendations to be made for maximizing the anabolic response to exercise. [Lecture 12]

Arazi, Hamid, Arsalan Damirchi, Hassan Faraji, and Rahman Rahimi. "Hormonal Responses to Acute and Chronic Resistance Exercise in Middle-Age versus Young Men." *Sport Sciences for Health* 8, no. 2 (2012): 59–65. In this experiment, researchers examined responses of the endocrine system to moderate-resistance training in younger verses middle-aged men; the men participated in an eight-week moderate-resistance training program three times per week. [Lecture 19]

Arble, D. M., J. Bass, A. D. Laposky, M. H. Vitaterna, and F. W. Turek. "Circadian Timing of Food Intake Contributes to Weight Gain." *Obesity* 17, no. 11 (2009): 2100–2102. This study focuses on the role of the circadian phase of food consumption in weight gain. [Lecture 13]

Arciero, P. J., M. J. Ormsbee, C. L. Gentile, B. C. Nindl, J. R. Brestoff, and M. Ruby. "Increased Protein Intake and Meal Frequency Reduces Abdominal Fat during Energy Balance and Energy Deficit." *Obesity* 21, no. 7 (2013): 1357–1366. The effects of consuming traditional versus higher protein intakes as three or six meals per day on abdominal fat, postprandial thermogenesis, and cardiometabolic biomarkers in overweight individuals during 28 days of energy balance and deficit were compared in this study. [Lecture 9]

Bailey, Regan L., et al. "Dietary Supplement Use in the United States, 2003–2006." *Journal of Nutrition* 141, no. 2 (2011): 261–266. The purpose of this analysis was to estimate dietary supplement use using the NHANES 2003–2006. [Lecture 10]

Bar-Or, Oded. "The Juvenile Obesity Epidemic: Strike Back with Physical Activity." *Gatorade Sports Science Institute* 16, no. 2 (2003): 1–6. Available at http://www.gssiweb.org/Article/sse-89-the-juvenile-obesity-epidemic-strike-back-with-physical-activity. The focus of this article is on combatting juvenile obesity with exercise. [Lecture 1]

Bartlett, J., G. Close, and D. Maclaren. "High-Intensity Interval Running Is Perceived to Be More Enjoyable Than Moderate-Intensity Continuous Exercise: Implications for Exercise Adherence." *Journal of Sports Sciences* 29, no. 6 (2011): 547–553. The aim of this study was to objectively quantify ratings of perceived enjoyment using the Physical Activity Enjoyment Scale following high-intensity interval running versus moderate-intensity continuous running. [Lecture 17]

Bassett, D. R., J. A. Vachon, A. O. Kirkland, E. T. Howley, G. E. Duncan, and K. R. Johnson. "Energy Cost of Stair Climbing and Descending on the College Alumnus Questionnaire." *Medicine and Scence in Sports Exercise* 29, no. 9 (1997): 1250–1254. The goal of this study was to quantify the energy cost of stair climbing and stair descending by measuring oxygen uptake. [Lecture 16]

Bélisle, M., E. Roskies, and J. M. Lévesque. "Improving Adherence to Physical Activity." *Health Psychology* 6, no. 2 (1987): 159–172. This paper consists of two studies that tested the efficacy of Marlatt and Gordon's relapse-prevention approach in increasing attendance during an exercise program and continuation of exercise activities. [Lecture 21]

Berry, E. M. "Are Diets High in Omega-6 Polyunsaturated Fatty Acids Unhealthy?" *European Heart Journal Supplements* 3 (2001): D37–D41. This article reviews the connection between dietary omega-6 fatty acids and atherosclerosis, carcinogenesis, and insulin resistance. [Lecture 4]

Betts, J. A., J. D. Richardson, E. A. Chowdhury, G. D. Holman, K. Tsintzas, and D. Thompson. "The Causal Role of Breakfast in Energy Balance and Health: A Randomized Controlled Trial in Lean Adults." *The American Journal of Clinical Nutrition* 100, no. 2 (2014): 539–547. The aim of this study was to conduct a randomized controlled trial examining causal links between breakfast habits and all components of energy balance in free-living humans. [Lecture 3]

Blackburn, G. "Effect of Degree of Weight Loss on Health Benefits." *Obesity Research* 3 (1995): 211S–216S. This paper reviews the effect of degree of weight loss on specific disease states and risk factors and discusses the impact of ethnic background, fat distribution, age, and mode of weight loss on outcome. [Lecture 1]

Boirie, Y., M. Dangin, P. Gachon, M. P. Vasson, J. L. Maubois, and B. Beaufrère. "Slow and Fast Dietary Proteins Differently Modulate Postprandial Protein Accretion." *Proceedings of the National Academy of Sciences* 94, no. 26 (1997): 14930–14935. The speed of absorption of dietary amino acids by the gut varies according to the type of ingested dietary protein. [Lecture 13]

Børsheim, E., and R. Bahr. "Effect of Exercise Intensity, Duration, and Mode on Post-Exercise Oxygen Consumption." *Sports Medicine* 33, no. 14 (2003): 1037–1060. There are conflicting results regarding the recovery period after exercise and the excess postexercise oxygen consumption. [Lecture 17]

Brose, Andrea, Gianni Parise, and Mark A. Tarnopolsky. "Creatine Supplementation Enhances Isometric Strength and Body Composition Improvements Following Strength Exercise Training in Older Adults." *The Journals of Gerontology Series A: Biological Sciences and Medical Sciences* 58, no. 1 (2003): B11–B19. The goal was to determine whether creatine monohydrate supplementation would enhance the increases in strength and fat-free mass that develop during resistance exercise training in older adults. [Lecture 14]

Brouns, F., and W. Saris. "How Vitamins Affect Performance." *The Journal of Sports Medicine and Physical Fitness* 29, no. 4 (1989): 400–404. This study examined the impact of vitamins on exercise performance. [Lecture 10]

Burd, N. A., S. H. Gorissen, and L. J. C. van Loon. "Anabolic Resistance of Muscle Protein Synthesis with Aging." *Exercise and Sport Sciences Review* 41, no. 3 (2013): 169–173. The level of habitual physical activity might be fundamental to maintain the anabolic responsiveness to protein intake with aging. [Lecture 9]

Calton, Jayson B. "Prevalence of Micronutrient Deficiency in Popular Diet Plans." *Journal of the International Society of Sports Nutrition* 7 (2010): 1–9. Research has shown micronutrient deficiency to be scientifically linked to a higher risk of overweight/obesity and other dangerous and debilitating diseases. [Lecture 10]

Candow, Darren G., et al. "Effect of Whey and Soy Protein Supplementation Combined with Resistance Training in Young Adults." *International Journal of Sport Nutrition and Exercise Metabolism* 16, no. 3 (2006): 233–244. The purpose of this study was to compare changes in lean tissue mass, strength, and myofibrillar protein catabolism resulting from combining whey protein or soy protein with resistance training. [Lecture 12]

Cappuccio, F. P., et al. "Meta-Analysis of Short Sleep Duration and Obesity in Children and Adults." *Sleep* 31, no. 5 (2008): 619–626. This study was conducted to assess whether the evidence supports the presence of a relationship between short sleep duration and obesity at different ages and to obtain an estimate of the risk. [Lecture 22]

Chevion, Shlomit, et al. "Plasma Antioxidant Status and Cell Injury after Severe Physical Exercise." *Proceedings of the National Academy of Sciences* 100, no. 9 (2003): 5119–5123. This is a study of the effects of oxidative stress during strenuous exercise. [Lecture 4]

Clegg, M. E. "Medium-Chain Triglycerides Are Advantageous in Promoting Weight Loss although Not Beneficial to Exercise Performance." *International*

Journal of Food Sciences and Nutrition 61, no. 7 (2010): 653–79. This study reviews medium-chain triglycerdies for use with weight loss and exercise performance. [Lecture 23]

Costa, G. "The Problem: Shiftwork." *Chronobiology International* 14, no. 2 (1997): 89–98. Shift work, such as night work, causes disruption of biological rhythms and perturbation of the social and family life that can negatively affect performance efficiency, health, and social relations. [Lecture 13]

Dashti, Hassan S., et al. "Habitual Sleep Duration Is Associated with BMI and Macronutrient Intake and May Be Modified by CLOCK Genetic Variants." *American Journal of Clinical Nutrition* 10, no. 1 (2015): 135–143. Available at http://ajcn.nutrition.org/content/101/1/135.abstract. The objective of this study was to examine associations between habitual sleep duration, body mass index, and macronutrient intake and to assess whether CLOCK variants modify these associations. [Lecture 20]

Dattilo, M., et al. "Sleep and Muscle Recovery: Endocrinological and Molecular Basis for a New and Promising Hypothesis." *Medical Hypotheses* 77, no. 2 (2011): 220–222. Available at http://www.ncbi.nlm.nih.gov/pubmed/21550729. The authors hypothesized that sleep deprivation decreases the activity of protein synthesis pathways and increases the activity of degradation pathways, favoring the loss of muscle mass. [Lecture 20]

De Castro, J. M. "The Time of Day of Food Intake Influences Overall Intake in Humans." *Journal of Nutrition* 134, no. 1 (2004): 104–111. The hypothesis is that the time of day of food intake would be related to total intake such that intake early in the day would tend to reduce overall intake, whereas intake later in the day would tend to increase intake over the entire day. [Lecture 13]

De Zwaan, M., M. Burgard, and C. Schenck. "Night Time Eating: A Review of the Literature." *European Eating Disorders Review* 11, no. 1 (2003): 7–24. This study reviews the published research on nighttime eating, including the night eating syndrome and the nocturnal eating/drinking syndrome. [Lecture 13]

Dhurandhar, E. J., J. Dawson, A. Alcorn, L. H. Larsen, and E. A. Thomas, et al. "The Effectiveness of Breakfast Recommendations on Weight Loss: A Randomized Controlled Trial." *American Journal of Clinical Nutrition* 100, no. 2 (2014): 507–513. The authors tested the relative effectiveness of a recommendation to eat or skip breakfast on weight loss in adults trying to lose weight in a free-living setting. [Lecture 3]

Diepvens, Kristel, Klaas R. Westerterp, and Margriet S. Westerterp-Plantenga. "Obesity and Thermogenesis Related to the Consumption of Caffeine, Ephedrine, Capsaicin, and Green Tea." *American Journal of Physiology-Regulatory, Integrative and Comparative Physiology* 292, no. 1 (2007): R77–R85. Tools for obesity management—including caffeine, ephedrine, capsaicin, and green tea—have been proposed as strategies for weight loss and weight maintenance. [Lecture 14]

Donnelly, J. E., et al. "American College of Sports Medicine Position Stand. Appropriate Physical Activity Intervention Strategies for Weight Loss and Prevention of Weight Regain for Adults." *Medical Science and Sports Exercise* 41, no. 2 (2009): 459–471. The purpose of this study was to reexamine the evidence from 1999 to determine whether there is a level at which physical activity is effective for prevention of weight gain, weight loss, and prevention of weight regain. [Lecture 1]

Duckworth, A. L., C. Peterson, M. D. Matthews, and D. R. Kelly. "Grit: Perseverance and Passion for Long-Term Goals." *Journal of Personality and Social Psychology* 92, no. 6 (2007): 1087–1101. The authors tested the importance of the noncognitive trait called grit. [Lecture 21]

Duloo, A. G., J. Jacquet, and J. P. Montani. "How Dieting Makes Some Fatter: From a Perspective of Human Body Composition Autoregulation." *Proceedings of the Nutrition Society* 71, no. 3 (2012): 379–389. This paper attempts to address the plausibility and mechanistic basis by which dieting might predispose people to increased fatness. [Lecture 19, Lecture 22]

Fairfield, K., and R. Fletcher. "Vitamins for Chronic Disease Prevention in Adults." *The Journal of the American Medical Association* 287, no. 23

(2002): 3116–3126. Available at http://jama.jamanetwork.com/article. aspx?articleid=195038. This paper reviews the clinically important vitamins with regard to their biological effects, food sources, deficiency syndromes, potential for toxicity, and relationship to chronic disease. [Lecture 10]

Fielding, R. A. "Protein Nutrition Mediates Lean Body Mass Homeostasis in the Aging Warfighter." *Journal of Nutition* 143, no. 11 (2013): 1857S–1861S. This review highlights selective aspects of protein supplementation in older adults. [Lecture 9]

Figueroa, A., A. Wong, A. Kinsey, R. Kalfon, W. Eddy, and M. J. Ormsbee. "Effects of Milk Proteins and Combined Exercise Training on Aortic Hemodynamics and Arterial Stiffness in Young Obese Women with High Blood Pressure." *American Journal of Hypertension* 27, no. 3 (2014): 338–344. This paper examines the impact of milk proteins and combined exercise training on blood pressure, arterial function, and muscle strength. [Lecture 13]

Figueroa, Arturo, et al. "Effects of Diet and/or Low-Intensity Resistance Exercise Training on Arterial Stiffness, Adiposity, and Lean Mass in Obese Postmenopausal Women." *American Journal of Hypertension* (2013): 1–8. This study evaluates the independent and combined effects of a hypocaloric diet on pulse-wave velocity and body composition as well as low-intensity resistance exercise training with slow movement. [Lecture 18]

Fildes, A., J. Charlton, C. Rudisill, P. Littlejohns, A. T. Prevost, and M. C. Gulliford. "Probability of an Obese Person Attaining Normal Body Weight: Cohort Study Using Electronic Health Records." *American Journal of Public Health* 105, no. 9 (2015): e54–59. This paper examines the probability of an obese person attaining normal body weight. [Lecture 22]

Folch, N., et al. "Metabolic Response to a Large Starch Meal after Rest and Exercise: Comparison between Men and Women." *European Journal of Clinical Nutrition* 57, no. 9 (2003): 1107–1115. The authors hypothesize that net whole-body de novo lipogenesis could be larger in women than men and that glycogen and fat balance could be lower and higher, respectively, following a large pasta meal ingested after rest or exercise. [Lecture 6]

Folch, N., et al. "Metabolic Response to Small and Large 13C-Labelled Pasta Meals Following Rest or Exercise in Man." *British Journal of Nutrition* 85 (2001): 671–680. The metabolic response to a 150- or 400-gram 13C-labeled pasta meal was studied for eight hours following rest or exercise at low or moderate workload. [Lecture 6]

Ford, E. S., C. Li, A. G. Wheaton, D. P. Chapman, G. S. Perry, and J. B. Croft. "Sleep Duration and Body Mass Index and Waist Circumference among U.S. Adults." *Obesity* 22, no. 2 (2014): 598–607. Available at http://www.researchgate.net/publication/247772753_Sleep_Duration_and_Body_Mass_Index_and_Waist_Circumference_among_US_Adults. This paper aims to examine the form of the relationship between sleep duration and anthropometric measures and possible differences in these relationships by gender and race or ethnicity. [Lecture 13]

Foss, B., L. R. Saeterdal, O. Nordgard, and S. M. Dyrstad. "Exercise Can Alter Cortisol Responses in Obese Subjects." *Journal of Exercise Physiology* 17, no. 1 (2014): 67–77. The aim of this study was to examine the influence of a 22-week lifestyle intervention program on the cortisol response in 35 inactive, obese subjects. [Lecture 19]

Foster-Schubert, K. E., et al. "Effect of Diet and Exercise, Alone or Combined, on Weight and Body Composition in Overweight-to-Obese Post-Menopausal Women." *Obesity* 20, no. 8 (2012): 1628–1638. Available at http://www.ncbi.nlm.nih.gov/pmc/articles/PMC3406229/. The authors conducted a randomized trial among 439 overweight-to-obese postmenopausal sedentary women to determine the effects of a reduced-calorie, low-fat diet, a moderate facility-based aerobic exercise program, or the combination of both interventions, versus a no-lifestyle-change control on change in body weight and composition. [Lecture 24]

Frankenfield, D. C., et al. "Validation of Several Established Equations for Resting Metabolic Rate in Obese and Non-Obese People." *Journal of American Diet Association* 103, no. 9 (2003): 1152–1159. This research evaluates several equations for predicting resting metabolic rate against measured values in obese and nonobese people. [Lecture 15]

Garthe, I., et al. "Effect of Two Different Weight-Loss Rates on Body Composition and Strength and Power-Related Performance in Elite Athletes." *International Journal of Sport Nutrition and Exercise Metabolism* 21, no. 2 (2011): 97–104. Available at http://www.ncbi.nlm.nih.gov/pubmed/21558571. The aim of this study was to compare changes in body composition, strength, and power during a weekly body-weight loss of 0.7 percent slow reduction versus 1.4 percent fast reduction. [Lecture 24]

Gebel, K., et al. "Effect of Moderate to Vigorous Physical Activity on All-Cause Mortality in Middle-Aged and Older Australians." *Journal of the American Medical Association* 175, no. 6 (2015): 970–977. Available at http://archinte.jamanetwork.com/article.aspx?articleid=2212268. This paper examines whether the proportion of total moderate to vigorous physical activity (MVPA) that is achieved through vigorous activity is associated with all-cause mortality independently of the total amount of MVPA. [Lecture 17]

Geer, E. B., and W. Shen. "Gender Differences in Insulin Resistance, Body Composition, and Energy Balance." *Gender Medicine* 6, no. 1 (2009): 60–75. This review summarizes published data on gender differences in insulin resistance, body composition, and energy balance. [Lecture 19]

Gibala, M. "Molecular Responses to High-Intensity Interval Exercise." *Applied Physiology, Nutrition, and Metabolism* 34, no. 3 (2009): 428–432. This paper examines the plausibility that metabolic adaptations to high-interval endurance training could be mediated in part through signaling pathways that are normally associated with endurance training. [Lecture 17]

Goo, R. H., J. G. Moore, E. Greenberg, and N. P. Alazraki. "Circadian Variation in Gastric Emptying of Meals in Humans." *Gastroenterology* 93, no. 3 (1987): 515–518. This paper aims to determine whether gastric emptying could account for circadian changes. [Lecture 13]

Gortmaker, S. L., A. Must, A. M. Sobol, K. Peterson, G. A. Colditz, and W. H. Dietz. "Television Viewing as a Cause of Increasing Obesity among Children in the United States, 1986–1990." *Archives of Pediatrics and Adolescent Medicine* 150, no. 4 (1996): 356–362. This paper examines the relationship between hours of television viewed and the prevalence of overweight children in 1990 and the incidence and remission of overweight children from 1986 to 1990. [Lecture 1]

Greer, B. K., et al. "Branched-Chain Amino Acid Supplementation and Indicators of Muscle Damage after Endurance Exercise." *International Journal of Sports Nutrition and Exercise Metabolism* 17, no. 6 (2007): 595–607. The purpose of this study was to determine whether branched-chain amino acid supplementation attenuates indirect indicators of muscle damage during endurance exercise as compared with an isocaloric carbohydrate beverage or a noncaloric placebo beverage. [Lecture 8]

Groen, B. B. L., P. T. Res, B. Pennings, E. Hertle, J. M. G. Senden, W. H. M. Saris, and L. J. C. van Loon. "Intragastric Protein Administration Stimulates Overnight Muscle Protein Synthesis in Elderly Men." *American Journal of Physiology, Endocrinology, and Metabolism* 302 (2012): E52–60. This study focused on the impact of night feeding of protein on muscle protein synthesis in elderly men. [Lecture 9, Lecture 13]

Grün, Felix, and Bruce Blumberg. "Endocrine Disruptors as Obesogens." *Molecular and Cellular Endocrinology* 304, no. 1–2 (2009): 19–29. This review highlights recent advances in the understanding of the molecular targets and possible mechanisms of action for these compounds as well as areas of future research needed to evaluate the significance of their contribution to obesity. [Lecture 20]

———. "Minireview: The Case for Obesogens." *Molecular Endocrinology* 23, no. 8 (2009): 1127–1134. This review considers the evidence for obesogens, how they might act, and where future research is needed to clarify their relative contribution to the obesity epidemic. [Lecture 20]

Hamilton, M. T., et al. "Role of Low Energy Expenditure and Sitting in Obesity, Metabolic Syndrome, Type 2 Diabetes, and Cardiovascular Disease." *Diabetes* 56, no. 11 (2007): 2655–2667. The purpose was to examine the role of sedentary behaviors, especially sitting, on mortality, cardiovascular disease, type 2 diabetes, metabolic syndrome risk factors, and obesity. [Lecture 1]

Hartman, J. W., J. E. Tang, S. B. Wilkinson, M. A. Tarnopolsky, R. L. Lawrence, A. V. Fullerton, and S. M. Phillips. "Consumption of Fat-Free Fluid Milk after Resistance Exercise Promotes Greater Lean Mass Accretion Than Does Consumption of Soy or Carbohydrate in Young, Novice, Male Weightlifters." *American Journal of Clinical Nutrition* 86 (2007): 373–381. In this study, the effects of milk were compared to those of carbohydrate and soy after resistance exercise in young men. [Lecture 9, Lecture 12]

Haskell, W. L., et al. "Physical Activity and Public Health: Updated Recommendation for Adults from the American College of Sports Medicine and the American Heart Association." *Medicine & Science in Sports & Exercise* 39, no. 8 (2007): 1423–1434. In this article, the American College of Sports Medicine and the American Heart Association make recommendations for adults' physical activity and health. [Lecture 1]

Hoffman, Jay R., et al. "Effect of Protein-Supplement Timing on Strength, Power, and Body-Composition Changes in Resistance-Trained Men." *International Journal of Sport Nutrition* 19, no. 2 (2009): 172–185. The effect of 10 weeks of protein-supplement timing on strength, power, and body composition was examined in 33 resistance-trained men. [Lecture 12]

Hoffman, Jay, et al. "Effect of Creatine and ß-Alanine Supplementation on Performance and Endocrine Responses in Strength/Power Athletes." *International Journal of Sport Nutrition and Exercise Metabolism* 16, no. 4 (2006): 430–446. The effects of creatine and creatine plus beta-alanine on strength, power, body composition, and endocrine changes were examined during a 10-week resistance training program in collegiate football players. [Lecture 14]

Holt, S. H., et al. "An Insulin Index of Foods: The Insulin Demand Generated by 1000-kJ Portions of Common Foods." *American Journal of Clinical Nutrition* 66, no. 5 (1997): 1264–1276. The aim of this study was to systematically compare postprandial insulin responses to isoenergetic 1000-kilojoule (240-kilocalorie) portions of several common foods. [Lecture 6]

Holtcamp, Wendee. "Obesogens: An Environmental Link to Obesity." *Environmental Health Perspectives* 120, no. 2 (2012): a62–a68. Available at http://www.ncbi.nlm.nih.gov/pmc/articles/PMC3279464/. According to this research, obesogens might have a link to obesity. [Lecture 20]

Houston, D. K., B. J. Nicklas, J. Ding, T. B. Harris, and F. A. Tylavsky, et al. "Dietary Protein Intake Is Associated with Lean Mass Change in Older, Community-Dwelling Adults: The Health, Aging, and Body Composition (Health ABC) Study." *American Journal of Clinical Nutrition* 87 (2008): 150–155. The objective of the study was to determine the association between dietary protein and changes in total lean mass and nonboneappendicular lean mass in older, community-dwelling men and women. [Lecture 9]

Isacco, L., P. Duche, D. Thivel, A. Meddahi-Pelle, S. Lemoine-Morel, M. Duclos, and N. Boisseau. "Fat Mass Localization Alters Fuel Oxidation during Exercise in Normal Weight Women." *Medicine & Science in Sports & Exercise* 45, no. 10 (2013): 1887–1896. The purpose of this study was to investigate the effect of low- and high-abdominal to lower-body fat mass ratio on metabolic and hormonal responses during exercise in premenopausal normal-weight women. [Lecture 19]

Ivy, J. L. "Glycogen Resynthesis after Exercise: Effect of Carbohydrate Intake." *International Journal of Sports Medicine*, 19 (1998): S142–S145. This research analyzes how much carbohydrate to ingest after exercise and the effect on glycogen storage. [Lecture 12]

Josse, A. R., S. A. Atkinson, M. A. Tarnopolsky, and S. M. Phillips. "Increased Consumption of Dairy Foods and Protein during Diet- and Exercise-Induced Weight Loss Promotes Fat Mass Loss and Lean Mass Gain in Overweight and Obese Premenopausal Women." *Journal of Nutrition* 141 (2011): 1626–34. The hypothesis of this paper is that participants that consume a high-protein, high-milk-product diet will lose a larger ratio of fat mass to lean body mass than participants consuming an adequate protein diet with moderate or low dairy products during an intervention with energy restriction and an exercise routine. [Lecture 9]

Jówko, Ewa, et al. "Creatine and β-Hydroxy-β-Methylbutyrate (HMB) Additively Increase Lean Body Mass and Muscle Strength during a Weight-Training Program." *Nutrition* 17, no. 7 (2001): 558–566. This paper investigates whether creatine and β-hydroxy-β-methylbutyrate act by similar or different mechanisms to increase lean body mass and strength in humans undergoing progressive resistance exercise training. [Lecture 14]

Kalergis, M., A. Schiffrin, R. Gougeon, P. J. Jones, and J. F. Yale. "Impact of Bedtime Snack Composition on Prevention of Nocturnal Hypoglycemia in Adults with Type 1 Diabetes Undergoing Intensive Insulin Management Using Lispro Insulin before Meals: A Randomized, Placebo-Controlled, Crossover Trial." *Diabetes Care* 26, no. 1 (2003): 9–15. The aim of this paper was to determine the impact of four bedtime snack compositions on nocturnal glycemic control, including frequency of hypoglycemia and morning hyperglycemia, in adults with type 1 diabetes using lispro insulin before meals and NPH insulin at bedtime. [Lecture 13]

Katayose, Y., M. Tasaki, H. Ogata, Y. Nakata, K. Tokuyama, and M. Satoh. "Metabolic Rate and Fuel Utilization during Sleep Assessed by Whole-Body Indirect Calorimetry." *Metabolism* 58, no. 7 (2009): 920–926. sThe purpose of this study was to examine metabolic rate and substrate oxidation during sleep in relation to time of sleep and sleep stage. [Lecture 13]

Katzmarzyk, Peter, et al. "Sitting Time and Mortality from All Causes, Cardiovascular Disease, and Cancer." *Medicine & Science in Sports & Exercise* 41, no. 5 (2009): 998–1005. Researchers examined sitting time and mortality in a representative sample of 17,013 Canadians 18–90 years of age. [Lecture 1]

Keesey, R. E., and M. D. Hirvonen. "Body Weight Set-Points: Determination and Adjustment." *Journal of Nutrition* 127, no. 9 (1997): 1875S–1883S. It appears that hypothalamic mechanisms play a primary role in setting the level at which individuals regulate body weight, and it is likely that the genetic, dietary, and other lifespan influences on body weight are expressed through these mechanisms. [Lecture 22]

Kerksick, Chad, et al. "Journal of the International Society of Sports Nutrition Position Stand: Nutrient Timing." *Journal of the International Society of Sports Nutrition* 5 (2008): 17. The position of the society regarding nutrient timing and the intake of carbohydrates, proteins, and fats in reference to healthy, exercising individuals is summarized by eight points. [Lecture 12]

Kern, Ben D., and Tracey L. Robinson. "Effects of β-Alanine Supplementation on Performance and Body Composition in Collegiate Wrestlers and Football Players." *The Journal of Strength & Conditioning Research* 25, no. 7 (2011): 1804–1815. The purpose of this study was to examine the effectiveness of beta-alanine as an ergogenic aid in tests of anaerobic power output after eight weeks of high-intensity interval, repeated sprint, and resistance training in previously trained collegiate wrestlers and football players. [Lecture 14]

Kinsey, A. W., W. R. Eddy, T. A. Madzima, L. B. Panton, P. J. Arciero, J. S. Kim, and M. J. Ormsbee. "Influence of Night-Time Protein and Carbohydrate Intake on Appetite and Cardiometabolic Risk in Sedentary Overweight and Obese Women." *British Journal of Nutition* 112 (2014): 320–327. This study focused on the acute effect of nighttime feeding in overweight women. [Lecture 9, Lecture 13]

Knab, A. M., et al. "A 45-Minute Vigorous Exercise Bout Increases Metabolic Rate for 14 Hours." *Medicine & Science in Sports & Exercise* 43, no. 9 (2011): 1643–1648. This study investigated the effects of inserting a 45-minute vigorous cycling bout into the daily schedule versus a controlled resting day on 24-hour energy expenditure in a metabolic chamber. [Lecture 17]

Koball, A. M., M. R. Meers, A. Storfer-Isser, S. E. Domoff, and D. R. Musher-Eizenman. "Eating When Bored: Revision of the Emotional Eating Scale with a Focus on Boredom." *Health Psychology* 31, no. 4 (2012): 521–524. This study explored whether eating when bored is a distinct construct from other negative emotions by revising the emotional eating scale to include a separate boredom factor. [Lecture 21]

Koopman, R., L. Verdijk, R. J. F. Manders, A. P. Gijsen, M. Gorselink, E. Pijpers, A. J. M. Wagenmakers, and L. J. C. van Loon. "Co-Ingestion of Protein and Leucine Stimulates Muscle Protein Synthesis Rates to the Same Extent in Young and Elderly Lean Men." *American Journal of Clinical Nutrition* 84, no. 3 (2006): 623–632. This paper investigates the effects on whole-body protein balance and mixed-muscle protein synthesis rates of the ingestion of carbohydrate with or without protein and free leucine after simulated activities of daily living. [Lecture 9]

Kouri, E. M., H. G. Pope Jr., D. L. Katz, and P. Oliva. "Fat-Free Mass Index in Users and Nonusers of Anabolic-Androgenic Steroids." *Clinical Journal of Sport Medicine* 5, no. 4 (1995): 223–228. This paper calculated fat-free mass index in a sample of 157 male athletes, comprising 83 users of anabolic-androgenic steroids and 74 nonusers. [Lecture 2]

Kravitz. L. "Research Sheds New Light on the Exercise 'Afterburn.'" *IDEA Fitness Journal* April (2015): 16–18. Available at http://www.unm.edu/~lkravitz/Article%20folder/ExerciseAfterburn2015.html. Recent research studies help clarify the body's ability to keep burning extra calories long after we stop exercising. [Lecture 17]

Laufs, U., S. Wassmann, T. Czech, T. Münzel, M. Eisenhauer, M. Böhm, and G. Nickenig. "Physical Inactivity Increases Oxidative Stress, Endothelial Dysfunction, and Atherosclerosis." *Arteriosclerosis, Thrombosis, and Vascular Biology* 25, no. 4 (2005): 809–814. Sedentary lifestyle is associated with increased cardiovascular events; the underlying molecular mechanisms are incompletely understood. [Lecture 4]

Lee, T. K., I. J. Clarke, J. St. John, I. R. Young, and B. L. Leury, et al. "High Cortisol Responses Identify Propensity for Obesity That Is Linked to Thermogenesis in Skeletal Muscle." *The FASEB Journal* 28, no. 1 (2014): 35–44. Predisposition to obesity can be predicted by cortisol responsiveness to an adrenocorticotropin challenge, and the response is due to innate differences in muscle thermogenesis. [Lecture 19]

Libotte, E., et al. "The Influence of Plate Size on Meal Composition: Literature Review and Experiment." *Appetite* 82 (2014): 91–96. Available at http://www.sciencedirect.com/science/article/pii/S0195666314003675. This study conducts a literature review and a controlled laboratory experiment to investigate whether plate size influences the composition of a meal and the total meal energy. [Lecture 20]

Madzima, T. A., L. B. Panton, S. K. Fretti, A. W. Kinsey, and M. J. Ormsbee. "Night-Time Consumption of Protein or Carbohydrate Results in Increased Morning Resting Energy Expenditure in Active College-Aged Men." *British Journal of Nutrition* 111 (2014): 71–77. This study focused on the acute effect of nighttime feeding in fit young men. [Lecture 9, Lecture 13]

Mastorakos, G., M. Pavlatou, E. Diamanti-Kandarakis, and G. P. Chrousos. "Exercise and the Stress System." *Hormones* 4, no. 2 (2005): 73–89. There is increasing incidence of exercise-related short-term and long-term consequences on female reproduction. [Lecture 19]

Meredith, C. N., et al. "Dietary Protein Requirements and Body Protein Metabolism in Endurance-Trained Men." *Journal of Applied Physiology* 66, no. 6 (1989): 2850–2856. This study examined endurance runners and nitrogen balance to understand protein needs. [Lecture 8]

Micha, R., and D. Mozzaffarian. "Saturated Fat and Cardiometabolic Risk Factors, Coronary Heart Disease, Stroke, and Diabetes: A Fresh Look at the Evidence." *Lipids* 45, no. 10 (2010): 893–905. Available at http://www.ncbi.nlm.nih.gov/pubmed/20354806. Researchers reviewed the evidence from randomized controlled trials of lipid and non-lipid risk factors, prospective cohort studies of disease endpoints, and disease endpoints for cardiometabolic effects of saturated fatty acid consumption in humans. [Lecture 7]

Michalakis, K., D. G. Goulis, A. Vazaiou, G. Mintziori, A. Polymeris, and A. Abrahamian-Michalakis. "Obesity in the Ageing Man." *Metabolism: Clinical and Experimental* 62, no. 10 (2013): 1341–1349. The aim of this narrative review is to present and discuss the current evidence on the changes in body composition, energy balance, and endocrine environment that occur in the aging man. [Lecture 19]

Miller, M. A., and R. H. Rahe. "Life Changes Scaling for the 1990s." *Journal of Psychosomatic Research* 43, no. 3 (1997): 279–292. In this study, varying influences of gender, age, marital status, and education were explored in more detail. [Lecture 21]

Miller, Paige E., and Vanessa Perez. "Low-Calorie Sweeteners and Body Weight and Composition: A Meta-Analysis of Randomized Controlled Trials and Prospective Cohort Studies." *The American Journal of Clinical Nutrition* 100, no. 3 (2014): 765–777. Available at http://ajcn.nutrition.org/content/early/2014/06/18/ajcn.113.082826.full.pdf+html. The objective of this study was to systematically review and quantitatively evaluate randomized controlled trials and prospective cohort studies, separately, that examined the relation between low-calorie sweeteners and body weight and composition. [Lecture 20]

Misner, B. "Food Alone May Not Provide Sufficient Micronutrients for Preventing Deficiency." *Journal of the International Society of Sports Nutrition* 3, no. 1 (2006): 51–55. The American Dietetic Association has stated that the best nutritional strategy for promoting optimal health and reducing the risk of chronic disease is to wisely choose a wide variety of foods, but this paper aims to show that this is not the only way. [Lecture 10]

Mozaffarian, R. S., et al. "Identifying Whole Grain Foods: A Comparison of Different Approaches for Selecting More Healthful Whole Grain Products." *Public Health Nutrition* 16, no. 12 (2013): 2255–2264. This paper investigates how five recommended whole grain criteria relate to healthfulness and price of grain products. [Lecture 11]

Murphy, C. H., T. A. Churchward-Venne, C. J. Mitchell, N. M. Kolar, and A. Kassis, et al. "Hypoenergetic Diet-Induced Reductions in Myofibrillar Protein Synthesis Are Restored with Resistance Training and Balanced Daily Protein Ingestion in Older Men." *American Journal of Physiology, Endocrinology, and Metabolism* 308, no. 9 (2015): E734–743. This article is about the way dietary protein distribution affects muscle protein syntheis. [Lecture 9]

National Institutes of Health and National Heart, Lung, and Blood Institute. "Clinical Guidelines on the Identification, Evaluation, and Treatment of Overweight and Obesity in Adults." Obesity Education Initiative. Available at http://www.nhlbi.nih.gov/guidelines/obesity/ob_gdlns.pdf. These are guidelines from the National Institutes of Health and the National Heart, Lung, and Blood Institute on how to identify, evaluate, and treat obesity. [Lecture 1]

Nigg, C. R., B. Borrelli, J. Maddock, and R. K. Dishman. "A Theory of Physical Activity Maintenance." *Journal of Applied Psychology* 57 (2008): 544–560. This paper presents the physical activity maintenance theory, which incorporates individual psychosocial variables (goal setting, motivation, and self-efficacy) and contextual variables of the environment and life stress (triggers of relapse). [Lecture 21]

Ormsbee, M. J., A. W. Kinsey, W. R. Eddy, T. A. Madzima, P. J. Arciero, A. Figueroa, and L. B. Panton. "The Influence of Nighttime Feeding of Carbohydrate or Protein Combined with Exercise Training on Appetite and Cardiometabolic Risk in Young Obese Women." *Applied Physiology in Nutrition and Metabolism* 40 (2015): 37–45. This study examined the additive impact of nighttime feeding of whey, casein, or carbohydrate combined with exercise training on appetite, cardiometabolic health, and strength in obese women. [Lecture 9, Lecture 13]

Ormsbee, Michael J., et al. "Fat Metabolism and Acute Resistance Exercise in Trained Men." *Journal of Applied Physiology* 102, no. 5 (2007): 1767–1772. The purpose of this study was to investigate the effect of acute resistance exercise on lipolysis within adipose tissue and subsequent substrate oxidation to better understand how resistance exercise might contribute to improvements in body composition. [Lecture 18]

Ormsbee, Michael J., et al. "Regulation of Fat Metabolism during Resistance Exercise in Sedentary Lean and Obese Men." *Journal of Applied Physiology* 106, no. 5 (2009): 1529–1537. The effect of acute resistance exercise on whole-body energy expenditure and α_2-adrenergic receptor regulation of lipolysis in subcutaneous abdominal adipose tissue was determined in sedentary lean and obese men. [Lecture 18]

Ormsbee, Michael J., et al. "The Effects of Six Weeks of Supplementation with Multi-Ingredient Performance Supplements and Resistance Training on Anabolic Hormones, Body Composition, Strength, and Power in Resistance-Trained Men." *Journal of International Society of Sports Nutrition* 9, no. 1 (2012): 49. The purpose of this study was to investigate the impact of specific pre- and post-workout multi-ingredient performance supplements on anabolic hormones, body composition, muscle strength, and power in resistance-trained men participating in a periodized resistance training program. [Lecture 14, Lecture 18]

Pagoto, Sherry L., and Bradley M. Appelhans. "A Call for an End to the Diet Debates." *The Journal of the American Medical Association* 310 (2013): 687–688. Available at http://jama.jamanetwork.com/article. aspx?articleid=1730520. The results of this study showed that adherence is the key to any dietary intervention. [Lecture 23, Lecture 24]

Paoli, et al. "High-Intensity Interval Resistance Training (HIRT) Influences Resting Energy Expenditure and Respiratory Ratio in Non-Dieting Individuals." *Journal of Translational Medicine* 10 (2012): 237. The authors tested the acute effects of high-intensity interval resistance training versus traditional resistance training on resting energy expenditure and respiratory ratio at 22 hours after exercise. [Lecture 17]

Park, S. K., et al. "The Effect of Combined Aerobic and Resistance Exercise Training on Abdominal Fat in Obese Middle-Aged Women." *Journal of Physiological Anthropology and Applied Human Science* 22, no. 3 (2003): 129–135. This study investigated the effect of both aerobic and resistance exercise on fat loss. [Lecture 1]

Pasiakos, S. M., J. J. Cao, L. M. Margolis, E. R. Sauter, and L. D. Whigham, et al. "Effects of High-Protein Diets on Fat-Free Mass and Muscle Protein Synthesis Following Weight Loss: A Randomized Controlled Trial."

Federation of American Societies for Experimental Biology 27 (2013): 3837–3847. This study measured the effects of high-protein diets on muscle mass after weight loss. [Lecture 1, Lecture 9]

Paul, G. L. "The Rationale for Consuming Protein Blends in Sports Nutrition." *Journal of the American College of Nutrition* 28, no. 4 (2009): 464S–472S. This review focuses on the potential nutritional advantages of combining whey protein, casein, and isolated soy protein. [Lecture 13]

Pelley, Janet. "Plasticizer May Make Boys Less Masculine." *Environmental Science and Technology*. November 12, 2008. This study measured the environmental impact on hormones that influence body composition. [Lecture 20]

Pietiläinen, K. H., S. E. Saarni, J. Kaprio, and A. Rissanen. "Does Dieting Make You Fat? A Twin Study." *International Journal of Obesity* 36, no. 3 (2012): 456–464. The objective of this study is to investigate whether the paradoxical weight gain associated with dieting is better related to genetic propensity to weight gain than to the weight-loss episodes themselves. [Lecture 19, Lecture 22]

Pope, Zachary K., Jeffrey M. Willardson, and Brad J. Schoenfeld. "Exercise and Blood Flow Restriction." *The Journal of Strength & Conditioning Research* 27, no. 10 (2013): 2914–2926. The purpose of this review was to discuss the relevant literature with regard to the type and magnitude of acute responses and chronic adaptations associated with blood flow restriction exercise protocols versus traditional non–blood flow restriction exercise protocols. [Lecture 18]

Prabhakaran, B., et al. "Effect of 14 Weeks of Resistance Training on Lipid Profile and Body Fat Percentage in Premenopausal Women." *British Journal of Sports Medicine* 33, no. 3 (1999): 190–195. The objective of this study was on the effects of a supervised, intensive (85 percent of one-repetition maximum) 14-week resistance training program on lipid profile and body fat percentage in healthy, sedentary, premenopausal women. [Lecture 1]

Raalte, J., W. Brewer, B. Lewis, D. Linder, G. Wildman, and J. Kozimor. "Cork! The Effects of Positive and Negative Self-Talk on Dart Throwing Performance." *Journal of Sport Behavior* 18 (1995): 50–57. The effects of positive and negative self-talk on dart-throwing performance were studied. [Lecture 21]

Reinehr, T. "Obesity and Thyroid Function." *Molecular and Cellular Endocrinology* 316, no. 2 (2010): 165–171. This is a study on thyrotropin and obesity. [Lecture 19]

Ren, R., X. Jiang, X. Zhang, Q. Guan, C. Yu, Y. Li, L. Gao, H. Zhang, and J. Zhao. "Associations between Thyroid Hormones and Body Fat in Euthyroid Subjects." *Clinical Endocrinology* 80, no. 4 (2014): 585–590. The aim of this study was to explore the association between thyroid hormones and body fat in a euthyriod population. [Lecture 19]

Renaud, H. J., J. Y. Cui, H. Lu, and C. D. Klaassen. "Effect of Diet on Expression of Genes Involved in Lipid Metabolism, Oxidative Stress, and Inflammation in Mouse Liver: Insights into Mechanisms of Hepatic Steatosis." *PloS one* 9, no. 2 (2014): e88584. This study examined the molecular changes elicited by nine diets with varying fat, sugar, cholesterol, omega-3 fatty acids, omega-6 fatty acids, and calories in C57BL/6 male mice. [Lecture 4]

Res, P. T., B. Groen, and B. Pennings, et al. "Protein Ingestion before Sleep Improves Postexercise Overnight Recovery." *Medicine & Science in Sports & Exercise* 44, no. 8 (2012): 1560–1569. This paper assessed the effect of protein ingestion immediately before sleep on digestion and absorption kinetics and protein metabolism during overnight recovery from a single bout of resistance-type exercise. [Lecture 13]

Riera-Crichton, D., and N. Tefft. "Macronutrients and Obesity: Revisiting the Calories In, Calories Out Framework." *Economics and Human Biology* 14 (2014): 33–49. Available at http://www.ncbi.nlm.nih.gov/pubmed/?term=Mac ronutrients+and+obesity%3A+Revisiting+the+calories+in%2C+calories+out +framework. The authors conducted dynamic time series and structural vector autoregressions analyses of U.S. data between 1974 and 2006 and a panel analysis of 164 countries between 2001 and 2010. [Lecture 1, Lecture 11]

Roberts, Justin D., et al. "The Effect of a Decaffeinated Green Tea Extract Formula on Fat Oxidation, Body Composition and Exercise Performance." *Journal of the International Society of Sports Nutrition* 12 (2015): 1–9. The aim of this study was to determine whether a decaffeinated green tea extract positively influenced fat oxidation, body composition, and exercise performance in recreationally active participants. [Lecture 14]

Roef, G., B. Lapauw, S. Goemaere, H. G. Zmierczak, K. Toye, and J. M. Kaufman. "Body Composition and Metabolic Parameters Are Associated with Variation in Thyroid Hormone Levels among Euthyroid Young Men." *European Journal of Endocrinology* 167, no. 5 (2012): 719–726. The authors investigated the relationship between thyroid hormone concentrations and body composition with metabolic parameters in a population of healthy euthyroid men. [Lecture 19]

Rognmo, Øivind, et al. "Cardiovascular Risk of High- versus Moderate-Intensity Aerobic Exercise in Coronary Heart Disease Patients." *Circulation* 126, no 12 (2012): 1436–1440. Available at http://www.ncbi.nlm.nih.gov/pubmed/22879367. The authors examined the risk of cardiovascular events during organized high-intensity interval exercise training and moderate-intensity training among 4,846 patients with coronary heart disease in three Norwegian cardiac rehabilitation centers. [Lecture 17]

Romon, M., C. Boulenguez, and P. Frimat. "Circadian Variation of Diet-Induced Thermogenesis." *American Journal of Clinical Nutrition* 57, no. 4 (1993): 476–480. The objective of this study was to assess a circadian variation of diet-induced thermogenesis that could favor weight gain among night workers used to eating a nighttime snack. [Lecture 13]

Santalla, A., C. P. Earnest, J. A. Marroyo, and A. Lucia. "The Tour de France: An Updated Physiological Review." *International Journal of Sports Physiology and Performance* 7 (2012): 200–209. The purpose of this brief review is to summarize what is currently known of the physiological demands of the Tour de France as well as of the main physiological profile of Tour de France competitors. [Lecture 12]

Schoenfeld, Brad Jon, Alan Albert Aragon, and James W. Krieger. "The Effect of Protein Timing on Muscle Strength and Hypertrophy: A Meta-Analysis." *Journal of International Society of Sports Nutrition* 10 (2013): 1–13. The purpose of this paper was to conduct a multilevel meta-regression of randomized controlled trials to determine whether protein timing is a viable strategy for enhancing postexercise muscular adaptations. [Lecture 12]

Schoenfeld, Brad J., et al. "Influence of Resistance Training Frequency on Muscular Adaptations in Well-Trained Men." *Journal of Strength and Conditioning Research* 29, no. 7 (2015): 1821–1829. The purpose of this study was to investigate the effects of training muscle groups one day per week using a split-body routine versus three days per week using a total-body routine on muscular adaptations in well-trained men. [Lecture 18]

Schroeder, E. Todd, et al. "Are Acute Post-Resistance Exercise Increases in Testosterone, Growth Hormone, and IGF-1 Necessary to Stimulate Skeletal Muscle Anabolism and Hypertrophy?" *Medicine & Science in Sports & Exercise* 45, no. 11 (2013): 2044–2051. This paper aims to support that post–resistance exercise increases in certain hormones are "optimal" for maximizing skeletal muscle anabolism and hypertrophy. [Lecture 18]

Schuler, Lou. "Protein: The Manual for Men." *Men's Health.* August 2015. Available at http://www.menshealth.com/meat. This is a guide on meat and health for men. [Lecture 18]

Schutz, Y., U. U. Kyle, and C. Pichard. "Fat-Free Mass Index and Fat Mass Index Percentiles in Caucasians Aged 18–98 Years." *International Journal of Obesity and Related Metabolic Disorders* 26, no. 7 (2002): 953–60. The purpose of this study was to determine reference values for fat-free mass index and fat mass index in a large Caucasian group of apparently healthy subjects, as a function of age and gender and to develop percentile distribution for these two parameters. [Lecture 2]

Simopoulos, A. P. "The Importance of the Ratio of Omega-6/Omega-3 Essential Fatty Acids." *Biomedical and Pharmaceutical* 56, no. 8 (2002):

365–379. Available at http://www.ncbi.nlm.nih.gov/pubmed/12442909. This study analyzed fish oil components and why they are important. [Lecture 7]

Skinner, Tina L., et al. "Factors Influencing Serum Caffeine Concentrations Following Caffeine Ingestion." *Journal of Science and Medicine in Sport* 17, no. 5 (2014): 516–520. The purpose of this paper is to determine whether differences in training status, body composition, and/or habitual caffeine intake influenced serum caffeine concentrations following caffeine ingestion. [Lecture 14]

Skinner, Tina L., et al. "Influence of Carbohydrate on Serum Caffeine Concentrations Following Caffeine Ingestion." *Journal of Science and Medicine in Sport* 16, no. 4 (2013): 343–347. The purpose of this paper is to examine the effect of a high-carbohydrate meal on serum caffeine concentration following caffeine intake. [Lecture 14]

Snijders, T., J. S. Smeets, S. van Vliet, J. van Kranenburg, and K. Maase, et al. "Protein Ingestion before Sleep Increases Muscle Mass and Strength Gains during Prolonged Resistance-Type Exercise Training in Healthy Young Men." *The Journal of Nutrition* (2015). This paper assessed the impact of dietary protein supplementation before sleep on muscle mass and strength gains during resistance-type exercise training. [Lecture 13]

Spear, B. A. "Does Dieting Increase the Risk for Obesity and Eating Disorders?" *Journal of the American Dietetic Association* 106, no. 4 (2006): 523–525. This study examines how dieting might contribute to disordered eating. [Lecture 19]

Stetson, B., A. O. Beacham, S. J. Frommelt, K. N. Boutelle, J. D. Cole, C. H. Ziegler, and S. W. Looney. "Exercise Slips in High-Risk Situations and Activity Patterns in Long-Term Exercisers: An Application of the Relapse Prevention Model." *Annals of Behavioral Medicine* 30, no. 1 (2005): 25–35. The purpose of this study was to examine the relationships among characteristics of exercise high-risk situations, components of the relapse prevention model relevant to exercise slips, and follow-up exercise outcomes in long-term community exercisers. [Lecture 21]

Stunkard, A., R. Berkowitz, T. Wadden, C. Tanrikut, E. Reiss, and L. Young. "Binge Eating Disorder and the Night-Eating Syndrome." *International Journal of Obesity and Related Metabolic Disorders* 20, no. 1 (1996): 1–6. The purpose of this study was to determine in three samples of obese women the prevalence of two eating disorders: binge eating disorder and the night-eating syndrome. [Lecture 13]

Sumithran, P., et al. "Long-Term Persistence of Hormonal Adaptations to Weight Loss." *New England Journal of Medicine* 365, no. 17 (2011): 1597–1604. This paper attempts to figure out the reasons behind the high rate of weight regain after diet-induced weight loss. [Lecture 22]

Symons, T. B., S. E. Schutzler, T. L. Cocke, D. L. Chinkes, R. R. Wolfe, and D. Paddon-Jones. "Aging Does Not Impair the Anabolic Response to a Protein-Rich Meal." *American Journal of Clinical Nutrition* 86, no. 2 (2007): 451–456. Available at http://www.ncbi.nlm.nih.gov/pubmed/17684218. This paper aims to characterize changes in plasma amino acid concentrations and to quantify muscle protein synthesis in healthy young people and elderly people after ingestion of a 113-gram (4-ounce) serving of lean beef. [Lecture 9]

Tang, J. E., D. R. Moore, G. W. Kujbida, M. A. Tarnopolsky, and S. M. Phillips. "Ingestion of Whey Hydrolysate, Casein, or Soy Protein Isolate: Effects on Mixed Muscle Protein Synthesis at Rest and Following Resistance Exercise in Young Men." *Journal of Applied Physiology* 107, no. 3 (2009): 987–992. This study was designed to compare the acute response of mixed muscle protein synthesis to rapidly and slowly digested proteins both at rest and after resistance exercise. [Lecture 9]

Tarnopolsky, M. A., et al. "Evaluation of Protein Requirements for Trained Strength Athletes." *Journal of Applied Physiology* 73, no. 5 (1992): 1986–1995. Leucine kinetic and nitrogen balance methods were used to determine the dietary protein requirements of strength athletes compared with sedentary subjects. [Lecture 8]

Thomas, D. M., et al. "Can a Weight Loss of One Pound a Week Be Achieved with a 3500-Kcal Deficit? Commentary on a Commonly Accepted Rule."

International Journal of Obesity (London) 37, no. 12 (2013): 1611–1613. In this paper, the authors demonstrate the risk of applying the 3,500-kilocalorie rule even as a convenient estimate by comparing predicted against actual weight loss in seven weight-loss experiments conducted in confinement under total supervision or objectively measured energy intake. [Lecture 14]

Thorpe, L. E., et al. "Prevalence and Control of Diabetes and Impaired Fasting Glucose in New York City." *Diabetes Care* 32, no. 1 (2009): 57–62. The purpose of the study was to determine the prevalence of diabetes and impaired fasting glucose and to assess clinical management indicators among adults with diabetes in a representative sample of New York City adults. [Lecture 1]

Thunders, M., S. Mangai, and R. Cooper. "Nutrigenetics, Nutrigenomics, and the Future of Dietary Advice." *Food and Nutrition Sciences* 4, no. 10 (2013): 999–1003. We might need a simpler approach to health care, one that embraces genetic variation yet focuses on the optimum nutritional benefit of dietary components. [Lecture 4]

Tieland, M., K. J. Borgonjen-Van den Berg, L. J. C. van Loon, and L. C. P. G. M. de Groot. "Dietary Protein Intake in Community-Dwelling, Frail, and Institutionalized Elderly People: Scope for Improvement." *European Journal of Nutrition* 51, no. 2 (2012): 173–179. This paper assessed the dietary protein intake, distribution of protein intake throughout the day, and use of protein-containing food sources in community-dwelling, frail, and institutionalized elderly people in the Netherlands. [Lecture 9]

Timmerman, Gayle M., and Adama Brown. "The Effect of a Mindful Restaurant Eating Intervention on Weight Management in Women." *Journal of Nutrition Education and Behavior* 44, no. 1 (2012): 22–28. Available at http://www.jneb.org/article/S1499-4046%2811%2900264-8/abstract. The purpose of this study was to evaluate the effect of a mindful restaurant eating intervention on weight management. [Lecture 24]

Trapp, E. G., D. J. Chisholm, J. Freund, and S. H. Boutcher. "The Effects of High-Intensity Intermittent Training on Fat Loss and Fasting Insulin Levels of

Young Women." *International Journal of Obesity* 32, no. 4 (2008): 684–691. The purpose of this study was to determine the effects of a 15-week high-intensity intermittent exercise program on subcutaneous and trunk fat and insulin resistance of young women. [Lecture 16]

Van Cauter, E., D. Désir, C. Decoster, F. Féry, and E. O. Balasse. "Nocturnal Decrease in Glucose Tolerance during Constant Glucose Infusion." *Journal of Clinical Endocrinology and Metabolism* 69, no. 3 (1989): 604–611. Studies comparing glucose tolerance in the morning versus tolerance in the evening have suggested that the time of day might influence glucose regulation. [Lecture 13]

Veldhuis, J. D. "Changes in Pituitary Function with Ageing and Implications for Patient Care." *Nature Reviews Endocrinology* 9, no. 4 (2013): 205–215. The aim of this article is to critically discuss the mechanisms mediating clinical facets of changes in the hypothalamic-pituitary axis during aging and the extent to which confounding factors operate to obscure aging-related effects. [Lecture 19]

Volek, J. S., et al. "Low-Carbohydrate Diets Promote a More Favorable Body Composition Than Low-Fat Diets." *Strength & Conditioning Journal* 32, no. 1 (2010): 42–47. A low-carbohydrate diet with periodized resistance training promotes greater fat loss while preserving lean body mass and promotes improvements to metabolic health. [Lecture 23]

Wall, Benjamin T., et al. "Chronic Oral Ingestion of L–Carnitine and Carbohydrate Increases Muscle Carnitine Content and Alters Muscle Fuel Metabolism during Exercise in Humans." *The Journal of Physiology* 589, no. 4 (2011): 963–973. The authors determined the effects of chronic l-carnitine and carbohydrate ingestion on muscle total carnitine content and exercise metabolism and performance in humans. [Lecture 14]

Waller, S. M., J. S. Vander Wal, and D. M. Klurfeld, et al. "Evening Ready-to-Eat Cereal Consumption Contributes to Weight Management." *Journal of the American College of Nutrition* 23, no. 4 (2004): 316–321. This study tested the hypothesis that providing a structured snack in the form of a "ready-to-eat" breakfast cereal would help regulate excess energy intake and contribute to weight loss in night snackers. [Lecture 13]

Weigle, D. S. "Appetite Regulation of Body Composition." *Federation of American Societies for Experimental Biology* 8, no. 3 (1994): 302–310. The implications of this adipose tissue–related satiety factor for the pathogenesis of obesity and the possible nature of the factor are discussed within this paper. [Lecture 22]

Werle, C. O. C., B. Wansink, and C. Payne. "Is It Fun or Exercise? The Framing of Physical Activity Biases Subsequent Snacking." *Marking Letters* (2014): 1–12. This paper offers the simple advice to consumers to make certain that they make their physical activity routine fun in order to avoid compensation. [Lecture 22]

Willis, L. H., C. A. Slentz, L. A. Bateman, A. T. Shields, and L. W. Piner, et al. "Effects of Aerobic and/or Resistance Training on Body Mass and Fat Mass in Overweight or Obese Individuals." *Journal of Applied Physiology* 113, no. 12 (2012): 1831–1837. Available at http://www.ncbi.nlm.nih.gov/pubmed/23019316. Researchers compared the effects of similar amounts of aerobic and resistance training on body mass and fat mass in overweight adults. [Lecture 17]

Wilmore, J. H., E. R. Buskirk, EM. DiGirolamo, and T. G. Lohman. "Body Composition: A Round Table." *The Physician and Sports Medicine* 14, no. 3 (1986): 144–162. Four experts assess body fat levels. [Lecture 2]

Wilson, Jacob M., et al. "The Effects of 12 Weeks of Beta-Hydroxy-Beta-Methylbutyrate Free Acid Supplementation on Muscle Mass, Strength, and Power in Resistance-Trained Individuals: A Randomized, Double-Blind, Placebo-Controlled Study." *European Journal of Applied Physiology* 114, no. 6 (2014): 1217–1227. This paper investigated the effects of 12 weeks of beta-hydroxy-beta-methylbutyrate supplementation on skeletal muscle hypertrophy, body composition, strength, and power in trained individuals. [Lecture 14]

Wroblewski, Andrew P., et al. "Chronic Exercise Preserves Lean Muscle Mass in Masters Athletes." *Physician and Sportsmedicine* 39, no. 3 (2011): 172–178. This study evaluated whether high levels of chronic exercise prevents the loss of lean muscle mass and strength experienced in sedentary aging adults. [Lecture 18]

Yang, Quanhe, et al. "Added Sugar Intake and Cardiovascular Diseases Mortality among U.S. Adults." *JAMA Internal Medicine* 174, no. 4 (2014): 516–524. The authors observed a significant relationship between added sugar consumption and increased risk for cardiovascular disease mortality. [Lecture 6]

Yang, Y., L. Breen, N. A. Burd, A. J. Hector, and T. A. Churchward-Venne, et al. "Resistance Exercise Enhances Myofibrillar Protein Synthesis with Graded Intakes of Whey Protein in Older Men." *British Journal of Nutrition* 108, no. 10 (2012): 1780–1788. This study aimed to determine the dose response of myofibrillar protein synthesis with the ingestion of isolated whey protein, with and without prior resistance exercise, in the elderly. [Lecture 9]

Image Credits

Page 4: © designer491/iStock/Thinkstock.

Page 8: © Monkey Business Images/Shutterstock.

Page 15: © wavebreakmedia/Shutterstock.

Page 17: © sssimone/iStock/Thinkstock.

Page 22: © Syda Productions/Shutterstock.

Page 32: © morisfoto/iStock/Thinkstock.

Page 41: © Syda Productions/Shutterstock.

Page 46: © Elena Schweitzer/Shutterstock.

Page 54: © Subbotina Anna/Shutterstock.

Page 57: © tiverylucky/Shutterstock.

Page 61: © alexpro9500/Shutterstock.

Page 66: © Daxiao Productions/Shutterstock.

Page 71: © Alexander Lukatskiy/Shutterstock.

Page 76: © Syda Productions/Shutterstock.

Page 80: © 13Smile/Shutterstock.

Page 84: © Pat_Hastings/Shutterstock.

Page 88: © wavebreakmedia/Shutterstock.

Page 91: © Mike Flippo/Shutterstock.

Page 97: © Eugenio Marongiu/Shutterstock.

Page 104: © Anna Omelchenko/Shutterstock.

Page 107: © InesBazdar/Shutterstock.

Page 112: © Valentyn Volkov/Shutterstock.

Page 115: © Africa Studio/Shutterstock.

Page 123: © Lilyana Vynogradova/Shutterstock.

Page 128: © Kaspars Grinvalds/Shutterstock.

Page 132: © lzf/Shutterstock.

Page 136: © Syda Productions/Shutterstock.

Page 139: © l i g h t p o e t/Shutterstock.

Page 144: © VectorLifestylepic/Shutterstock.

Page 155: © Image Point Fr/Shutterstock.

Page 158: © Monika Wisniewska/Shutterstock.

Page 163: © Yuriy Rudyy/Shutterstock.

Page 171: © Andrey_Popov/Shutterstock.

Page 174: © Andresr/Shutterstock.

Page 182: © catsinside/iStock/Thinkstock.

Page 187: © nito/Shutterstock.

Page 194: © Ditty_about_summer/Shutterstock.

NOTES

NOTES

NOTES

NOTES

NOTES

NOTES